DYSTHYMIA AND THE SPECTRUM
OF CHRONIC DEPRESSIONS

DYSTHYMIA
AND THE SPECTRUM
OF CHRONIC DEPRESSIONS

Hagop S. Akiskal
Giovanni B. Cassano
Editors

THE GUILFORD PRESS
New York   London

© 1997 The Guilford Press
A Division of Guilford Publications, Inc.
72 Spring Street, New York, NY 10012

Printed in the United States of America

This book is printed on acid-free paper.

Last digit is print number: 9 8 7 6 5 4 3 2 1

Library of Congress Cataloging-in-Publication Data

Dysthymia and the spectrum of chronic depressions / Hagop S.
  Akiskal, Giovanni B. Cassano, editors.
      p. cm.
    Includes bibliographical references and index.
    ISBN 1-57230-089-2
    1. Depression, Mental.   I. Akiskal, Hagop S.   II. Cassano,
G. B. (Giovanni B.)
    [DNLM: 1. Depression, Mental.   2. Dysthymic Disorder.
3. Chronic Disease.   WM 171 D9975 1997]
RC537.D97 1997
61.85′27—dc21
DNLM/DLC   97-11003
for Library of Congress   CIP

Contributors

HAGOP S. AKISKAL, MD, Department of Psychiatry, International Mood Center, University of California at San Diego, La Jolla, California

JULES ANGST, MD, Research Department, Psychiatric University Hospital, Zurich, Switzerland

GIOVANNI B. CASSANO, MD, Institute of Clinical Psychiatry, School of Medicine, University of Pisa, Pisa, Italy

JONATHAN R. T. DAVIDSON, MD, Anxiety and Traumatic Stress Program, Department of Psychiatry, Duke University Medical Center, Durham, North Carolina

DONNA B. GREENBERG, MD, Department of Psychiatry, Massachusetts General Hospital, Harvard Medical School, Boston, Massachusetts

DANIEL N. KLEIN, PhD, Department of Psychology, State University of New York at Stony Brook, Stony Brook, New York

DONALD F. KLEIN, MD, Department of Therapeutics, New York State Psychiatric Institute, New York, New York; Department of Psychiatry, College of Physicians and Surgeons, Columbia University, New York, New York

RACHEL G. KLEIN, PhD, Department of Clinical Psychology, New York State Psychiatric Institute, New York, New York; Department of Psychiatry, College of Physicians and Surgeons, Columbia University, New York, New York

JAMES H. KOCSIS, MD, Department of Psychiatry, New York Hospital–Cornell Medical Center, New York, New York

MARIA KOVACS, PhD, Department of Psychiatry, Western Psychiatric Institute and Clinic, University of Pittsburgh School of Medicine, Pittsburgh, Pennsylvania

YVON D. LAPIERRE, MD, Departments of Psychiatry and Pharmacology, University of Ottawa, Ottawa, Ontario, Canada

MARIO MAJ, MD, Departments of Medicine and Surgery, Institute of Psychiatry, University of Naples, Naples, Italy

ANDREAS MARNEROS, MD, Psychiatric Hospital, University of Bonn, Bonn, Germany

GREGORY A. MILLER, PhD, Department of Psychology, University of Illinois, Champaign–Urbana, Illinois

STUART A. MONTGOMERY, MD, Department of Pharmacology, Imperial College of Medicine at St. Mary's, University of London, London, United Kingdom

C. Q. MOUNTJOY, MD, St. Andrew's Hospital, Northampton, Northampton, United Kingdom

A. EGIDIO NARDI, MD, Anxiety and Depression Research Program, Institute of Psychiatry, Federal University of Rio de Janeiro, Rio de Janeiro, Brazil

ARUN V. RAVINDRAN, MD, University of Ottawa, Ottawa, Ontario, Canada; Institute of Mental Health Research, Royal Ottawa Hospital, Ottawa, Ontario, Canada

ANKE ROHDE, MD, Section on Psychosomatics in Gynecology, University of Bonn, Bonn, Germany

SIR MARTIN ROTH, MD, Department of Surgery, University of Cambridge Clinical School, Cambridge, United Kingdom

MARIO SAVINO, MD, Institute of Clinical Psychiatry, University of Pisa, Pisa, Italy

JONATHAN W. STEWART, MD, Department of Psychiatry, College of Physicians and Surgeons, Columbia University, New York, New York; Department of Therapeutics, New York State Psychiatric Institute, New York, New York

MARCIO VERSIANI, MD, Anxiety and Depression Research Program, Institute of Psychiatry, Federal University of Rio de Janeiro, Rio de Janeiro, Brazil

Preface

Yet none despair is mild
Even as the winds and waters are;
I could lie down like a tired child,
And weep away this life of care
Which I have borne, and yet must bear,
Till death like sleep might steal on me . . .
Breathe o'er my dying brain in last monotony.
—P. B. SHELLEY (*lines written in dejection,*
near Naples, 1818)

Shelley is testimony that even mild melancholy is difficult to bear: Four years after he wrote this Neapolitan poem of dejection, he was found drowned off the coast of Portovenere, in Northern Italy. This book is about the suffering of those who must bear depression over long periods of time, often over a lifetime.

Chronic depressive disorders are increasingly commanding the attention of psychiatrists, clinical psychologists, and social workers, as well as physicians in primary care settings. Traditionally considered forms of "character" or "neurotic" depressive pathology, during the past decade there has been a paradigmatic shift of thinking and research that emphasizes affective origin for a significant proportion of patients suffering from these disorders. This shift, in turn, has had a revolutionary impact on how these disorders are clinically managed; in particular, innovative psychopharmacological approaches have been creatively applied in the treatment of dysthymia and many other chronic depressive conditions that were previously deemed beyond biology. This volume documents these far-reaching changes in our thinking about the nature and treatment of these conditions. The chapters that constitute this book derive, in part, from an international symposium that took place in Spoleto, Italy, on April 24–25, 1992, and critically examined the clinical and therapeutic significance of these changes. The meeting was held under the auspices of the Italian Psychiatric Association and was made possible through an unrestricted grant from Eli Lilly Italia. All chapters have been exclusively edited and updated, and several chapters, not presented at the meeting, were specifically written for this volume.

This book opens with an overview of chronic depressions and continues with six chapters on officially sanctioned chronic affective rubrics such as dysthymia, chronic major depression, and residual depressive states. These chapters are followed by reviews on the classic—now officially discarded—construct of neurotic depression, present-day neurasthenias, and atypical depressions. The next three chapters consider the unofficial rubrics of hysteroid dysphoria and recurrent brief depressions. The final two chapters deal with issues of chronicity of depressive and conduct disorders arising in childhood. Thus, the book covers the entire spectrum of chronic depressive conditions encountered in clinical practice.

The volume progresses logically from current official diagnostic concepts and their classical roots to newly proposed chronic depressive rubrics. We have attempted to preserve much of the lively atmosphere of debate that prevailed during the Spoleto meeting. Thus, although readers can discern several broad areas of consensus on chronic depressions, we have avoided uniformity of views. In particular, we have given visibility to diverse concepts and research developed in Europe, the Americas, and Japan. Chapters represent state-of-the-art reviews on the clinical features and treatment of chronic depressive conditions. However, given the paucity of systematic psychotherapy studies in chronic depressions, no chapter has been specifically assigned to this topic. Chronic depression represents a new focus of clinical investigation and therapeutics, and this volume is presented to the field as a summary of current findings that can serve as stimulus for further research. Certainly, long-term studies need to be conducted, and, in particular, psychosocial approaches geared to the problems of chronic depressives and their families should receive greater research attention.

Above all, as academic researchers who practice psychiatry, we have endeavored to make the volume both data-based *and* relevant to the practice needs of clinicians. We believe this to be the primary mission of clinical departments of universities. We feel this statement of purpose is warranted by the fact that the complexity of contemporary clinical challenges of chronic mental illness facing our field appears to have driven many young and senior colleagues into the "safer" retreat of either administration or "pure" research. We offer this volume as one possible antidote: Greater understanding of the causes and successful clinical management of chronic depressive disorders will lessen the suffering of the patients and the burden on their families, as well as the countertransference that often leads to defensive avoidance of such patients as severe, intractable "character" disorders. Finally, we submit this volume as a definitive shift of the theory and practice in the realm of chronic depressive conditions from an era dominated by art to one of increasingly sophisticated clinical science. This new paradigm in the field of chronic depressions can be enhanced if practitioners adopt the stance of clinician–researcher, utilizing a systematic approach to the evaluation and treatment of the clinical challenges posed by their chronically depressive patients.

HAGOP S. AKISKAL
GIOVANNI B. CASSANO

Contents

CHAPTER 1   Overview of Chronic Depressions and Their   1
Clinical Management
Hagop S. Akiskal

CHAPTER 2   Dysthymia: Clinical Picture, Comorbidity, and Outcome   35
Marcio Versiani
A. Egidio Nardi

CHAPTER 3   Primary Dysthymia: Predictors of Treatment Response   44
Arun V. Ravindran
Yvon D. Lapierre

CHAPTER 4   Chronic and Residual Major Depressions   54
Giovanni B. Cassano
Mario Savino

CHAPTER 5   Chronic Depression: The Efficacy of Pharmacotherapy   66
James H. Kocsis

CHAPTER 6   "Residual States" in Affective, Schizoaffective,   75
and Schizophrenic Disorders
Andreas Marneros
Anke Rohde

CHAPTER 7   Depressive Personality: Relationship to Dysthymia   87
and Major Depression
Daniel N. Klein
Gregory A. Miller

CHAPTER 8   The Need for the Concept of Neurotic Depression   96
Martin Roth
C. Q. Mountjoy

CHAPTER 9   A Critical Reappraisal of the Concept of Neurotic Depression   130
Mario Maj

CHAPTER 10 Beyond Neurasthenia and Chronic Fatigue   148
Donna B. Greenberg

CHAPTER 11 Atypical Depressions   165
Jonathan R. T. Davidson

CHAPTER 12 Chronic (and Hysteroid) Dysphorias   174
Jonathan W. Stewart
Donald F. Klein

CHAPTER 13 Minor and Recurrent Brief Depression   183
Jules Angst

CHAPTER 14 Suicide in Chronic and Recurrent Depressions   191
Stuart A. Montgomery

CHAPTER 15 Depression and Attention-Deficit/Hyperactivity Disorder   198
Rachel G. Klein

CHAPTER 16 Chronic Depression in Childhood   208
Maria Kovacs

Index   221

CHAPTER 1

Overview of Chronic Depressions and Their Clinical Management

Hagop S. Akiskal

Chronic and intermittent depressive conditions today represent a large proportion of patients seen by mental health specialists. Though typically of low-grade intensity, these depressions, nonetheless, produce cumulative impairment due to the protracted course of the affective pathology (Keller, 1994). Astute clinical observers (e.g., Kraines, 1957) have always been aware of protracted depressions, yet only recently these conditions seem to be more prevalent in clinical settings, thereby posing logistic, diagnostic, and therapeutic challenges. Their increasing current visibility in tertiary care and research settings is in part because more classical episodic depressions are being taken care of by generalists in both the general health and mental health sectors. Moreover, the availability of new treatments for mood disorders has destigmatized depression, and, as a consequence, an increasing number of individuals with low-grade, "minor" and/or "atypical" symptoms or course are seeking relief for their suffering. Finally, both clinicians and epidemiologists have been increasingly willing to subsume these conditions under a broadened rubric of mood disorders.

Following a brief historical discussion of unofficial chronic depressive diagnostic concepts, this chapter focuses on dysthymic and partially remitted depressive disorders, both of which have been formally endorsed by the latest editions of the diagnostic manuals of the American Psychiatric Association (APA) and World Health Organization (WHO). This chapter, which is updated from previous reviews (Akiskal, 1991, 1992b; Akiskal &

1

Weise, 1992), focuses on clinical and therapeutic aspects of the greatest relevance to the practitioner.

The Misdiagnosis of Chronic Depressions

In the days before the third edition of the *Diagnostic and Statistical Manual of Mental Disorders* (DSM-III; APA, 1980), mood disorders were strictly considered episodic illnesses. This view was based on a misapprehension of Kraepelin's (1921) thesis that, in contrast to the deterioration observed in dementia praecox, manic–depressive conditions permitted return to the premorbid baseline. Kraepelin's more profound conceptualization postulated that affective episodes arose from the unstable baseline of temperamental disturbances. Kraepelin made use of the term "temperament" because of its biological connotation. Thus, temperaments—conceived as lifelong low-grade affective expressions—and superimposed full-blown affective episodes were both believed by Kraepelin to be of hereditary origin, hence "endogenous." Associated life circumstances and the interpersonal context were considered either incidental or provocative agents rather than causes. Recent collaborative research between the universities of Pisa and Tennessee tends to support Kraepelin's thesis (Musetti et al., 1989; Perugi et al., 1990; Cassano et al., 1992).

As long as psychiatry was hospital-based, the severe psychotic phases of depressive illness represented a radical departure from the patient's habitual temperament or personality. With the advent of outpatient psychiatry, clinicians were flooded with patients who presented with relatively milder depressive conditions; in these patients, the state of depression does not seem to represent a major departure from their habitual self or personality. This difficulty in separating low-grade depressives from their habitual selves meant that life disruptions and difficulties due to depression were not easily separable from events in their lives. All such patients had to do was to look into their past and blame some aspect of it as being "causative" of their depression, and psychosocially oriented clinicians were ready to believe them. Lacking the profound vegetative psychomotor disturbances and psychotic symptoms of hospitalized manic–depressive patients, chronic depressives were increasingly tagged with the "neurotic depressive" rubric (Akiskal et al., 1978). Their repetitive tendency to descend into gloomy despair was thus ascribed to an abnormal underlying personality reacting to relatively minor adversities in their lives. The primary illness of these patients was thereby believed to reside in their rigidity, hostile dependency, or histrionic, borderline, or psychopathic "characters" (Arieti & Bemporad, 1978). These considerations in turn explain why, until recently, neurotic depressions were not classified with the classical (episodic) mood disorders.

What emerges from the foregoing discussion is a picture of neurotic depression as a fluctuating illness based on the vagaries of the sufferer's character structure. Thus, some neurotic depressives could enjoy long periods of relatively normal life and then, faced with adversity, would crash into abject despair. Others would complain of dysphoria on an intermittent basis. In a still third group, persistently chronic gloomy mood characterizes the life course of the patient. Yet in all three instances, the depression is presumed to be "characterological" in origin. The usual argument presented in support for this characterological emphasis in formulating intermittent or chronic depressions ran something like this: Affective illness is classically episodic, representing a sharp break from one's usual self; personality disorder is chronic; chronic depression or disposition to repeated bouts of depression must therefore be secondary to personality disorder.

Prior to the mid-1980s, patients with chronic depression were the victims of such misguided clinical logic. Patients who could afford it were sentenced to the couch. These patients did not fare much better with psychopharmacologists, who generally ignored them, for fear that they would mess up the results of controlled antidepressant trials. Cognitive-behavioral researchers, too, generally avoided such patients for the same reason. That is why, until recently, the only clinicians who showed sustained interest in these chronic characterological depressions were those with psychodynamic bent (e.g., Arieti & Bemporad, 1978), the only group of clinicians not interested in results (at least in the short run)! Although these patients may have overall fared somewhat better in the hands of psychodynamic practitioners, they were typically tagged with character diagnoses (Bonime, 1966) reflecting the therapists' impotence to terminate the misery of these patients in the short term. Very few authors (e.g. Kraines, 1957; Klein, 1974; Akiskal, 1981; Cassano et al., 1983) emphasized the affective origin of chronic depression.

Neurotic Depressions and "Atypicality"

Although so-called neurotic depressions have higher prevalence in clinical practice today, they are often considered "atypical." Atypicality in this context refers to departure from the stereotype of the classical—more "typical"—endogenous type. Used in this informal sense, atypicality could actually mean different things (e.g., more chronic than episodic, minor (subsyndromal) as opposed to major (syndromal), anxious–lethargic rather than truly retarded). A more specific meaning of atypicality refers to "reverse vegetative signs" (i.e., evening worsening, initial insomnia, tendency to hypersomnolence, fatigue, and hyperphagia) (Davidson et al., 1982).

Although atypical, neurotic, or otherwise minor depressions are often contrasted to that of the "endogenous" subtype, several observations tend to raise reservations about the longitudinal validity of this distinction: (1) bipolar, especially bipolar II, depression often presents with atypical symptomatology (Himmelhoch et al., 1991); (2) such atypical "neurasthenic" presentations, followed prospectively, have been shown to precede bipolar illness (Akiskal et al., 1983; Ebert & Barocka, 1991); (3) family studies have shown that "endogenous" depressions do not breed true (Maier et al., 1992); (4) likewise, "minor" depressions cluster in the families of more classical depressives (Gershon et al., 1982; Maier et al., 1992). Such data are generally consistent with the viewpoint that what is transmitted in families are not specific depressive subtypes but general dimensions of depression, and that "atypicality" and "endogeneity" (as clinical constructs) do not refer to distinct affective disorders but represent alternative phases in the course of these disorders. That is why in the fourth edition of DSM (DSM-IV; APA, 1994) they are reserved to the status of qualifying phrases, just like "psychotic features," "seasonality," and "rapid cycling."

The foregoing position necessitates a general framework to explain the heterogeneity of clinical manifestations observed in depressive disorders. DSM-IV does not specifically provide such a framework. In my opinion, pathoplastic changes in the clinical picture of depression are a result of such factors as age and age at onset, gender, temperament, concurrent anxiety disorders, and/or substance abuse (Akiskal, 1983, 1992a). Furthermore, subcultural factors and objectively ascertainable aversive life situations could in selected instances so dominate the clinical picture of a depressive condition that they could pathoplastically color its manifestations.

Unfortunately, our current psychiatric nosology is most cogent in its description of the "typical" endogenous subtypes. Atypicality is often used as a negative definition for all those patients who deviate in significant ways from the endogenous prototype. What follows is a brief review of various nosological concepts—generally considered "minor" and/or nonendogenous—and which illustrate attempts to bring conceptual, clinical, and therapeutic definition to this large population (Akiskal & Weise, 1992). My intent is to illustrate how pathoplastic factors influence the clinical presentation of depression and to highlight the gradual shift of psychiatric thinking about these conditions from stress, neurotic, and characterological disorders to that of mood disorder.

Reactive Depressions

Classically these depressions are defined by the occurrence of a specific aversive life event. According to Jaspers (1962), (1) such a depression would not have occurred without the event (e.g., love loss) to which it is a reaction, (2) it will continue as long as the event is present, and (3) it would terminate with the reversal of the event (e.g., the return of the love object). Depressions meeting all three of these criteria are almost never seen in clinical practice. With interpersonal support, most people are able to face up to life reverses, which explains why reactive depressions are characteristically self-limiting. Therefore, reactive depressions are best considered adaptive responses or adjustment reactions.

Conceptually, however, it is possible to envision chronically unsatisfactory life situations which might engender chronic misery—and lead to "chronic reactive depression." This formulation remains controversial. Psychodynamic clinicians often raise the question, Why would an individual continue to stay in a painful life situation? And they sometimes evoke the concept of "masochism" to explain it (Simons, 1987). Such individuals are believed to be incapable of ridding themselves of painful life situations, the implication being that they somehow contribute to the maintenance of such painful situations. Neurotic conflicts implicit in this formulation might suggest the diagnosis of "chronic neurotic depression." Current research (see Widiger, 1987), however, suggests that many of these presumed "self-defeating" traits are perhaps more situation-specific than previously believed and might resolve with the elimination of the situation. So-called self-defeating features then are best conceptualized as psychodynamic mechanisms rather than being indicative of a specific personality. Klein's (1974) concept of chronic demoralization—describing individuals stuck in unresolvable life situations—actually better describes many of these patients than does chronic neurotic depression.

Anxious Depressions

This mixture of anxiety and depression refers to the simultaneous occurrence of anxious (e.g., the threat of loss) and depressive (e.g., the despair of loss) cognitions when confronted with a major life stressor (Akiskal, 1990a). This ongoing dynamic implies that the emotional disequilibrium progresses from anxiety to depression while the patient's mental state is still in flux, thereby explaining the subacute or chronic nature of the disorder. Despite recent research thrusts in this area, "anxious depression" is not an official diagnostic rubric. Its frequent use by clinicians and clinical researchers (Kendall & Watson, 1989, Maser & Cloninger, 1990), however, points to the almost universal presence of anxiety in depressive states, and especially its greater visibility when the depression is less prominent. Some authorities on both sides of the Atlantic argue that neurotic depressions arise as maladaptive response to anxiety and, on this etiological ground, suggest retaining the neurotic depressive rubric (Wolpe, 1988).

Recent preliminary genetic data (Kendler et al., 1992) indirectly tend to support the notion that certain depressive and generalized anxiety states are related. Indeed, Andrews et al. (1990) and Tyrer et al. (1992) have proposed that they belong to a common category of a "general neurotic syndrome." However, more research needs to be conducted in this area before unequivocally accepting such an entity as an official nosological rubric. The difficulty lies in the fact that, as currently defined, anxious depressions are extremely heterogeneous (Akiskal, 1990a). Thus, many endogenous depressives experience autonomic anxiety, tension, psychic anxiety, and dread of facing the day; it would be a mistake to consider them anxious depressives (Clayton et al., 1991; Coryell et al., 1992). Likewise, panic attacks, and intractable anxiety and tension are often part of the core pathology of mixed bipolar states in which dysphoria dominates the clinical picture (Akiskal & Mallya, 1987). Furthermore, various anxiety states often coexist with bipolar II (Savino et al., 1993). Finally, stimulant abuse or sedative-hypotic withdrawal could give rise to prominent anxiety manifestations in the setting of a major depressive illness (Van Valkenburg et al., 1984). Differentiating among these various possibilities has important implications for treatment and prognosis.

Neurasthenic and Related Conditions

The term "neurasthenia," which was coined more than 100 years ago by an American neuropsychiatrist, Beard (1881), refers to a more chronic stage of anxious–depressive symptomatology. The anxiety generated by overstress is so excessive that it is replaced by a chronic disposition to irritability, fatigue—especially mental fatigue—lethargy, and exhaustion. It is, as it were, that the sufferer's mind can no longer take on new stresses. A perusal of the clinical manifestations described by Beard shows that anxiety-related symptoms were preeminent in his time. These included, among others, headache, scalp tenderness, backache, heavy limbs, vague neuralgias, yawning, dyspepsia, palpitations, sweating hands and feet, chills, flushing, sensitivity to weather changes, insomnia, nightmares, pantaphobia, asthenopia, and tinnitus.

Although today the formal diagnosis of neurasthenia is more used in China than in the United States (Kleinman, 1986), the recent worldwide upsurge of popularity of the concept of chronic fatigue states attests to the clinical acumen of classic physicians. Despite much energy invested on a viral or immunological etiology, current descriptions tend to suggest an affective—anxiety or mood disorder—basis for many, but certainly not all, sufferers of this syndrome (Wessely, 1990; Greenberg, 1990). Like other patients presenting to primary care settings with somatic complaints, those with chronic fatigue tend to denounce psychiatric diagnoses as adequate explanations for their suffering.

Empathic listening might be a reasonable clinical approach to this difficult group of patients who are sometimes quite disabled. This would provide the practitioner with the opportunity to gather the necessary information to formulate an affective—or mixed anxious depressive—diagnosis which, in turn, would justify a vigorous trial of thymoleptic agents. The joint presence of several of the following features would lend support to such an approach: (1) fatigue is not alleviated by sleep or rest; (2) fatigue is worse in the morning; (3) such morning accentuation is part of a more generalized psychomotor inertia or lack of initiative; (4) fatigue is associated with anhedonia, including sexual anhedonia; (5) such fatigue, furthermore, coexists with anxious and pessimistic brooding; and (6) family history or past personal history for a more classical mood or anxiety disorder could be elicited with expert probing.

Atypical Depressions

Originally developed in England (West & Dally, 1959; Sargent, 1962), and currently under intense investigation at the New York Psychiatric Institute (Liebowitz et al., 1988) and at Duke (Davidson et al., 1982), the term "atypical" in its more specific connotation refers to fatigue superimposed on past history of somatic anxiety and phobias, together with "reverse vegetative signs" (mood worse in the evening, insomnia, tendency to oversleep and overeat). Given that nighttime sleep is disturbed in the first half of the night in many atypical depressives, irritability, hypersomnolence, and daytime fatigue might, in part, represent expected daytime stigmata of sleep deprivation due to intermittent initial insomnia (Akiskal & Lemmi, 1987). The temperament of these patients often consists of mood-reactive and rejection-sensitive traits, and there seems to be some specificity of the monoamine oxidase inhibitors (MAOIs) (and, possibly, serotonergic antidepressants) for these traits (see Davidson, Chapter 11; Stewart & Klein, Chapter 12, this volume). This is one of the main reasons why clinicians take the rubric of atypical depression seriously. This response profile seems to hold true even for those atypical patients experiencing the anergic depressive phase of bipolar illness (Himmelhoch et al.,

1991). Indeed, atypical depression might be the same as bipolar II disorder, or an alternative expression of it.

Hysteroid Dysphorias

As described by Liebowitz and Klein (1979), this concept refers to patients with atypical depression who additionally meet the following criteria: (1) giddy responses to romantic opportunities, and an avalanche of dysphoria (angry–depressive, even suicidal responses) upon romantic disappointment; (2) impaired anticipatory pleasure, yet perfectly capable of responding with pleasure when hedonic opportunities are offered by others (i.e., preservation of consummatory reward); and (3) craving for chocolate and sweets, which contain phenylethylamine compounds and/or sugars believed to facilitate cellular and neuronal intake of the amino-acid l-tryptophan, leading hypothetically to the brain's synthesis of endogenous antidepressants. Interestingly, the use of the adjective "hysteroid" was meant to convey that what appeared to be character pathology was in reality secondary to a biological disturbance in the substrates governing affect, drives, and reward. The hysteroid dysphorics' intense and unstable life suggests links to cyclothymia or bipolar II, a connection rarely made by the group of investigators who have developed the hysteroid dysphoria concept. This has obvious treatment implications beyond MAOIs. For instance, there might be considerable overlap with the "emotionally unstable character disorder"—studied earlier by the investigators from the same group (Rifkin et al., 1972)—and which is known to respond to small doses of chlorpromazine or lithium.

Characterological Depressions

This clinical colloquialism refers to patients with low-grade depression with intermittent fluctuating chronic course, thereby forming part of the sufferer's habitual self, such that it cannot be distinguished from his or her character structure. The characterological pathology is variously believed to represent a broad mélange of dependent, avoidant, passive–aggressive, histrionic, narcissistic, and borderline features. It is further believed that, in their attempt to obtain interpersonal rewards, such individuals bring on life situations that precipitate their depressive crashes. For many authorities these features represent the core pathology of neurotic depressions (Bonime, 1966). Curiously, there appears to be broad consensus on this point among authorities of both psychodynamic and neo-Kraepelinian persuasion. Parker and colleagues (1988) have expressed this position most eloquently in their inability to develop a clinical typology of neurotic depressions that excludes personality variables. Winokur (1987) has argued that these depressions are related—possibly genetically—to antisocial and related personality disorders in their first-degree relatives, many of whom also suffer from alcoholism; however, the Copenhagen adoption study of alcoholism (Goodwin et al., 1977) suggests an environmental factor (i.e., being raised by an alcoholic parent) to be responsible for such depressive-like character pathology. Whatever the origin of this pathology, emerging data—presented later in this chapter—suggest pharmacological responsivity in many such patients.

Brief Recurrent Depressions

This group of disorders has emerged largely from epidemiological work conducted in young cohorts in Zurich (Angst et al., 1990), as well as clinical studies on young patients with repeated suicide attempts studied in London (Montgomery et al., 1989). The description is that of short-lived depressions which recur on at least a monthly basis but are not menstrually related. They could coexist with major depression and dysthymia, even brief recurrent hypomania (Angst, 1992). Paradoxically, these European authors have been reluctant to draw parallels between brief recurrent depressions on the one hand and cyclothymic and soft bipolar disorders on the other (Akiskal, 1992b). Paskind (1929), who had described patients with brief episodes, classified them within the broad rubric of manic depression.

Brief recurrent depression is deemed to be rare in psychiatric settings: It has been suggested that it is more likely to be encountered in primary care settings. A more plausible explanation is that many psychiatrists are not accustomed to diagnose mood disorder in individuals with chronic-intermittent disorders, especially if the latter engage in repeated self-harm; such patients are more than likely mistakenly to be relegated to the realm of "borderline" character pathology.

The current nosological status of recurrent brief depressions is uncertain, but it testifies to Kraepelin's observation (1921) that many transitional forms link the depressive temperament to affective episodes of various duration, severity, and frequency of recurrence:

> A permanent gloomy stress in all the experiences of life . . . usually perceptible already in youth, and may persist without essential change throughout the whole of life . . . [or] there is actually an uninterrupted series of transitions to periodic melancholia . . . in which the course is quite indefinite with irregular fluctuations and remissions.

In this brief paragraph, Kraepelin postulates that some individuals exhibit lifelong tendencies toward gloom without developing episodes. He also describes various courses—persistent, intermittent, or episodic—intervening between the depressive temperamental disposition and full-blown affective illness. The importance of the concept of recurrent brief depression lies in that it provides an affective bridge between temperament (or the habitual self of the patient) and the more symptomatic (episodic or chronic) phases of the malady. The same appears to be the case for subsyndromal symptomatic depressions (Judd et al., 1994).

From Neurotic Depression to Dysthymia

DSM-III replaced the "neurotic depression" rubric with that of "dysthymic disorder" as a more accurate description of the long-standing pathology which predisposes to depression. At the same time, it classified dysthymia under mood disorders based on emerging evidence that neurotic character pathology reflected a more basic affective dysregulation (Akiskal et al., 1980; Rosenthal et al., 1981).

Shifting low-grade depressive pathology from the general category of neurosis to that of mood disorder represents a radical departure from traditional nosology. It is supported by prospective studies of neurotic depression (Akiskal et al., 1978; Bronisch et al., 1985) that demonstrated a recurrent unipolar or bipolar outcome in nearly 50%; others pursued a chronic or intermittent depressive course, and a significant minority were found to suffer from various anxiety and/or addictive disorders. Such heterogeneity of outcome and related considerations (Klerman et al., 1979) did necessitate eliminating neurotic depression from official nosology. Obviously, some neurotic depressions belong to the general class of anxiety and related disorders and were reclassified accordingly. Neurotic depressions were reclassified as major depressive or atypical bipolar disorders (atypical bipolar refers to the bipolar II subtype characterized by major depressive episodes and nonpsychotic elations), and the remainder—those pursuing a more chronic subsyndromal course—were subsumed under dysthymia.

Dysthymic disorder in DSM-III referred to all chronic depressions of two or more years. In DSM-III-R (APA, 1987) low-grade depressive states following major depressive episodes were distinguished from dysthymia proper, a disorder of insidious onset, low-grade severity, and chronic course. DSM-IV has essentially retained this distinction. Although in the current APA manual dysthymia can occur as a secondary complication of other psychiatric disorders, the core concept of dysthymia as conceptualized in Burton and Akiskal (1990) refers to a primary mood disorder with the following characteristics: (1) low-grade chronicity, for at least 2 years, which is not the sequel of a major depression; (2) not a complication in the course of a preexisting nonaffective psychiatric disorder; (3) insidious onset with origin often in childhood or adolescence; (4) persistent or intermittent course; and (5) ambulatory disorder, which is not incompatible with relatively "stable" functioning.

This stability though is precarious at best. Recent data from a series of studies have documented that many of these patients invest whatever "energy" they have in work, with none left for leisure and other family or social activities (Perugi et al., 1994), hence the marital friction so characteristic of their colorless lives, which appear to be overdedicated to work. These empirical findings on the dysthymics' "work orientation" echo earlier formulations on the melancholic type by Tellenbach (1980), who was himself undoubtedly influenced by Kraepelin's description (1921) of the depressive temperament: "Life with its activity is a burden which they habitually bear with dutiful self-denial without being compensated by the pleasures(s) of existence."

Chronicity does not imply presence of symptoms on a daily basis; intermittent symptoms are quite common. Furthermore, it is noteworthy that in DSM-III-R, personality disorder is considered to be present *concurrently* with dysthymia. This is an important change from DSM-III, which, despite its philosophy of considering personality disorders (Axis II) orthogonal to the major psychiatric syndromes (Axis I), contained the ambiguous statement that "often the affective features of [dysthymia] are viewed as secondary to an underlying personality disorder." DSM-IV has unfortunately reversed to an even more ambiguous conceptualization: While retaining dysthymia on Axis I, it has introduced a trait version of dysthymia—defined as an optional Axis II "depressive personality disorder." Depending on the clinical setting, as many as one out of three dysthymics might meet the criteria for such a personality (Klein, 1990). However, other dysthymics might exhibit avoidant, dependent, obsessive, narcissistic, historic, and even borderline features (Markowitz et al., 1992). The question then is whether anything has been achieved by the official APA classification substituting neurotic depression with dysthymia.

Dysthymia as a Subaffective Disorder

DSM-III had proposed the rubric of "dysthymia" for any chronic depression. Although this term (literally "ill-humored") has been broadly applied to all negative affective states with depressive, anxious, and obsessional qualities, the more classic connotation limits its use to subsyndromal and protracted depression (Akiskal, 1983). This was in part endorsed by

DSM-III-R, which restricted the operational territory of dysthymia to individuals with long-standing low-grade depressive suffering prior to superimposed depressive episodes, if any. Used in this sense, primary dysthymia refers to a basal condition: A dysthymic individual is one who is *habitually* lethargic, gloomy, brooding, incapable of fun, and preoccupied with personal inadequacy (Kraepelin, 1921; Kretschmer, 1936; Schneider, 1958). Despite significant overlap with its psychoanalytical analogue of depression-prone personality (Chodoff, 1972; Kernberg, 1986), the dysthymic temperament described in the German literature tends to deemphasize obsessionality, dependency, and masochism in favor of subdepressive traits. In the French literature this concept is reflected in what is termed *la dépression constitutionelle* (Peron-Magnan, 1992).

DSM-IV has retained dysthymia as a subsymptomatic construct on Axis II, at the same time raising the possibility that some dysthymics might also simultaneously meet the criteria for a trait diagnosis—that of depressive personality disorder. As discussed elsewhere (Akiskal, 1996), these dual symptomatological and trait definitions seem to represent alternative manifestations of a common constitutional depressive diathesis. ICD-10 (World Health Organization, 1992) seems closer to the mark when it suggests that dysthymia and depressive personality represent overlapping constructs.

What tends to confuse clinicians is that many dysthymic patients present clinically with significant personality pathology, and they have difficulty seeing an affective connection. The diagnostic and therapeutic dilemmas faced by practitioners in their clinical encounters may be related to the demanding nature of such patients and their almost exhibitionistic flaunting of suffering (Akiskal, 1983). Thus, chronically depressed patients who attended the University of Tennessee mood clinic have made statements such as, "I am a walking encyclopedia of depression," or, "I am the most miserable creature on earth." Such hyperbolic descriptions of suffering contrast so strongly with the relative absence of objectively ascertainable depression that these patients may understandably be considered "manipulative" or even "malingering." Many are nonassertive, but others are sarcastic, cynical, or nihilistic—attributes that can alienate the clinicians who care for them. Patients with an intellectual inclination may belabor themes of alienation and the absurdities of the human condition. Their *weltschmerz* ("weariness of life") may on occasion suggest "existential depression." Consideration of such issues, which may be initially alluring to even experienced therapists, often leads to a therapeutic impasse by diverting attention from the core affective pathology.

Although European psychiatry as far back as Hippocratic times conceptualized depressive personality attributes as "subclinical" expressions of affective disorder (von Zerssen, 1993), the North American position has been dominated by formulations that viewed milder depressions as derived from developmental vicissitudes (Arieti & Bemporad, 1978). Current evidence indicates that these vicissitudes themselves might represent the fact of being born to (an) affectively ill parent(s), with all the implied interactions, disruptions, and deprivations (Akiskal, 1986). Furthermore, depressive personality attributes—observed in prospective studies conducted on populations prior to the onset of clinical depression—are virtually impossible to separate from minor chronic depressive symptoms (Hirschfeld et al., 1989). Finally, as observed by Kraepelin and supported by current data, depressive personality traits tend to aggregate in the families of the affectively ill. These perspectives converge in suggesting that early onset dysthymia constitutes a subdepressive temperament. In this context, the term "temperament," as opposed to "personality" or "character," underscores closer link to an underlying affective biology. Actually, studies conducted on dysthymic children (see Kovacs, Chapter 16, this volume) have shown that this diagnosis is familially loaded with affective illness and predicts a highly recurrent course for superimposed major affective episodes (Kovacs et al., 1994). Such data, in turn, support the conceptualization of dysthymia as an early phenotype in the pathogenetic chain of affective illness (Akiskal, 1994a).

In some individuals, accounting for nearly 50% of dysthymics in the community (Robins & Regier, 1991), the illness does not progress beyond the temperamental or subsymptomatic stage. In those presenting clinically, superimposed episodes are observed in 80–90% (Akiskal, 1983). Thus, pure dysthymia is relatively uncommon in clinical practice; most mental health practitioners encounter dysthymia in its "double depressive" form (i.e., dysthymia with superimposed major depressive episodes) (Keller et al., 1983). The pure form of dysthymia might be more prevalent in private outpatient psychotherapy practice. Indeed, ICD-10 (World Health Organization, 1992) proposes to limit dysthymia to a chronic subthreshold depression which is only infrequently complicated by major depression of relatively mild intensity.

The symptom profile of dysthymia, as it has emerged from University of Tennessee research (Akiskal, 1990b), is summarized in Table 1.1. This profile obviously overlaps with that of major depression but differs from

TABLE 1.1. Core Symptomatology in Primary Dysthymia

Mood: gloomy, morose, brooding, anhedonic
Psychomotor: reticence, inertia, lethargy
Vegetative: diurnality (of any of the above)
Cognitive: low self-esteem, guilty ruminations, pessimistic
    outlook, thoughts of death

Note. Data from Akiskal (1990b).

it in that symptoms tend to outnumber signs. This translates into a more "subjective" than "objective" depression. Thus, marked disturbances in appetite and libido are uncharacteristic, and psychomotor agitation or retardation are not observed. Dysthymia then is depression with somewhat "muted" but chronic or intermittent symptomatology. Yet subtle "endogenous" features are commonly observed: psychomotor inertia, lethargy, and anhedonia, which are characteristically worse in the morning. Clinically, the striking features of dysthymia include habitual gloom, brooding, lack of *joie de vivre,* and preoccupation with inadequacy. Dysthymia then is best characterized as long-standing low-grade depression—experienced as part of the habitual self—and representing an accentuation of traits observed in the depressive temperament (see Table 1.2). Thus, dysthymia can be viewed as a more symptomatic form of this temperament. Sleep electroencephalographic data (Akiskal et al., 1980) indicate that many dysthymics exhibit the sleep patterns of acute major depressives, providing further support to the constitutional nature of the disorder.

Clinicians who adhere to the pre-DSM-III conceptualization of neurotic depression—which derived it from personality disorder—would generally assume that the proper management of such patients requires major psychotherapeutic effort in altering the pathological character structure. Clinicians who subscribe to the post-DSM-III conceptualization offered here—dysthymia considered as a subdepressive trait disorder—do not have the same degree of confidence in the necessity of a long-term investment in such effort; on the contrary, they point to evidence on the efficacy of thymoleptics in not only attenuating the affective symptoms (Howland, 1991) but even reversing much of the interpersonal disturbances (Kocsis et al., 1988; Stewart et al., 1988).

Despite much criticism for the substitution of neurotic depression by dysthymia on both sides of the Atlantic (see, for instance, Roth & Mountjoy, Chapter 8, this volume, on neurotic depression), it is its predictive validity with antidepressant pharmacotherapies that constitutes the most important argument in favor of dysthymia as a variant of primary affective illness (Burton & Akiskal, 1990). All nosological concepts are empty without such

TABLE 1.2. Attributes of the Depressive Temperament

Somber, humorless, and incapable of fun
Gloomy and brooding
Self-critical, self-reproaching, and guilt-prone
Preoccupied with inadequacy, failure, and pessimistic outcomes
Nonassertive, self-sacrificing, and devoted
Consider suffering as part of habitual self
Skeptical, hypercritical, and complaining

Note. Data from Akiskal (1983).

validity. Indeed, neurotic depression, its predecessor, can be indicted for its characterological connotations that tended to discourage competent pharmacotherapy. At least in North America, and selected centers in South America, the European continent and Japan, many psychiatrists have responded with clinical enthusiasm in treating the vast universe of "nonendogenous" intermittent or chronic depressives with pharmacotherapy. Kasahara (1991) and I (Akiskal, 1992a) have actually made treatment proposals of chronic depressive subtypes that depend on long-term traits rather then endogenous–neurotic symptom profiles. We believe this approach provides new hope for patients, and their families, with long-standing affective suffering previously deemed "refractory" to somatic interventions.

Residual Chronic Major Depression

In this section I consider another group of chronic depressives in which chronicity reflects residuals of incompletely remitted major depressive episodes.

The course of primary unipolar depressive illness beginning after age 50 is often protracted (Akiskal, 1982). Even in those patients with unremarkable premorbid history, in 15–20%, residual chronicity may develop after one or more depressive episodes fail to remit fully. During this residual phase, which may extend over several years, characterological manifestations—passivity, a sense of resignation, generalized fear of inability to cope, adherence to rigid routines, and inhibited communication—tend to dominate the clinical picture, with depressive symptoms pushed to the background. Marital conflict is often in a state of deadlock, with patients unable to divorce or to reconcile with their spouse. In other patients, the residual state is dominated by somatic manifestations involving vegetative or autonomic nervous system irregularities that mimic anxiety symptoms.

Weissman and Klerman (1977) have reported that failure to recover from depressive episodes is due to neuroticism, alcohol abuse, sedativism (often iatrogenic), and inadequate pharmacotherapy. The University of Tennessee study (Akiskal, 1982), which focused on primary depressives, found evidence for additional factors. First, we documented that rapid eye movement (REM) latency was shortened to less than 70 minutes on consecutive nights, not only during the acute episode but also during the chronic phase. This neurophysiological similarity suggested the value of conceptualizing the chronic phase as an affective process. This formulation was further reinforced by positive family history loaded for mood disorders in chronic depressives. Proximate stressors correlated with chronic outcome included disabled spouses, multiple losses of immediate family members through death, and concurrent disabling medical conditions such as rheumatologic, cardiovascular, or neurological diseases. Use of depressant antihypertensive agents and excessive use of alcohol and seda-tive–hypnotic agents were also prevalent in chronic depressives. These data overall suggest that multiple factors predispose patients to incomplete recovery from late onset primary major depressive episodes (Table 1.3). More recent studies by Scott (1988) and Musetti et al. (1989) support many of the Tennessee findings. Mueller et al. (1994) have confirmed alcoholism as a factor of chronicity in depression. In addition, Coryell et al. (1992) have found anxiety disorders to delay recovery from depression.

After removal of contributory pharmacological factors (e.g., depressant antihypertensives, benzodiazepines, or alcohol), most patients with residual depression can be satisfactorily managed with vigorous antidepressant pharmacotherapy. Although undertreatment continues to account for a proportion of residual chronicity in many depressed patients, recent clinical observations suggest that overzealous treatment with antidepressants—especially tricyclic antidepressants (TCAs)—might be the culprit in

TABLE 1.3. Comparison of 38 Chronic Primary Depressives (Mean Age 50.8 Years) with 40 Episodic Primary Depressive Controls (Mean Age 47 Years) on Selected Variables (Given in Percentages)

Variable	Chronic depressive	Episodic depressive	p^a
Female sex	76	80	ns
Family history			
Depression only	42	20	<.05
Bipolar illness	5	3	ns
Development			
Psychiatric illness in both parents	16	13	ns
Loss of parent < age 15	21	18	ns
Personality			
"Unstable"	21	16	ns
Depressive^b	44	28	ns
Stressors^c			
Multiple deaths in family	21	3	.033
Disabled family member	21	3	.033
Superimposed medical illness	47	10	.001
Use of depressant antihypertensives	21	3	.033
Secondary sedativism and alcoholism	34	17	.043

Note. Data from Akiskal (1982).

[a]Chi-square or Fisher's exact test.

[b]Based on criteria operationalized from Schneider (1958).

[c]Episodic group limited to 30 age- and sex-matched subjects.

a significant minority of patients. Thus, in some premorbidly hyperthymic individuals, continued TCA treatment of depressive episodes may lead not only to rapid cycling (Koukopulos et al., 1980; Wehr & Goodwin, 1987) but also to chronicity (Akiskal & Mallya, 1987). These highly dysphoric protracted residual states are characterized by unrelenting irritable mood; fatigue accompanied by racing thoughts; severe agitation, anxiety, and insomnia; unendurable sexual excitement despite the predominant negative affect; and an extroverted, seemingly "histrionic" demeanor accompanied nevertheless by genuine expressions of intense suffering. Clinically, such a symptomatological picture is best understood as a depressive state superimposed on a bipolar temperament that serves to generate the "soft" bipolar signs which, in turn, color the depressive picture with mixed features. The clinician should therefore note that the residual chronicity in some cases of recurrent depression in reality represents a protracted pseudo-unipolar mixed state. This nuance is of immense therapeutic relevance. These mixed residual states respond preferentially to lithium augmentation of the TCA regimen. In our experience, the method championed by de Montigny and colleagues (1981) is of little use with strictly unipolar patients and works best with this pseudo-unipolar group that exhibits "soft" signs of bipolarity (Akiskal et al., 1989). Carbamazepine, reportedly efficacious in some refractory depressions (Post et al., 1986) may do so for the same reason.

The foregoing considerations suggest that when a residual depression fails to respond adequately to vigorous antidepressant drug therapy, the physician should consider the possibility of either an underlying medical–neurological disease that renders the depression unresponsive to such therapy or a protracted mixed state arising from the substrate of a "soft bipolar" disorder for which traditional TCAs represent a hazard. Although selective serotonin reuptake inhibitors (SSRIs) are not entirely benign from this standpoint, clinically they seem quite efficacious for the entire spectrum of chronic depressions. Venlafaxine too appears efficacious on clinical grounds in refractory depressives. Nefazodone might be especially useful for those with prominent anxious symptomatology, and has the added advantage of absence of sexual side effects. Electroconvulsive therapy (ECT)—even maintenance ECT—should always be kept as an option in residual chronic depression.

Reticence to use ECT might underlie residual chronicity in many cases. In my experience, true refractoriness to pharmacotherapy occurs in less than 5% of chronic major depressives, which, in almost all cases, involves cryptic systemic or cerebral disease (Akiskal et al., 1989). When such disease is treatable (e.g., sleep apnea, nocturnal myoclonus, heart failure, endocrinopathies, Parkinson's disease), its amelioration with appropriate treatment would generally reduce the affective symptomatology.

Unfortunately, in rare cases the cryptic illness is an abdominal malignancy or malignant brain tumor discovered too late. Such considerations underscore the fact that clinicians treating chronic depressions must be astute to the possibility of underlying physical disease. One possible clinical clue to the existence of such disease is the development of atypical side effects to antidepressants (e.g., extreme hypersomnolence, agitation, or visual illusions) with extremely low doses of antidepressants.

Pharmacotherapy of Dysthymia

The reticence of many clinicians to use pharmacotherapy in alleviating the suffering of dysthymic patients derives in large part from the clinical presentations of this disorder. Insidious onset, dating back to late childhood or teens, and preceding superimposed major depressive episodes, if any, by years or even decades, characterizes the symptomatology of those chronically depressed patients most representative of the dysthymic patients. As a rule, patients return to the low-grade depressive pattern following recovery from superimposed episodes (Keller et al., 1983).

Such "residuals" might be misinterpreted as indicators of character pathology. Furthermore, patients with early onset dysthymia often speak of being "born depressed" or of being depressed "since conception" (Akiskal, 1983), and they seem to view themselves as belonging to an aristocracy of lifelong sufferers (Schneider, 1958). Such chronic dysphoria in the absence of observed signs of melancholia easily lends itself to the label of "characterological depression." This difficulty of separating the fluctuating course of depression from the patient's character structure is understandably reflected in diagnostic uncertainty and therapeutic impasse.

Pharmacological Dissection of Dysthymia

The Memphis studies conducted in the late 1970s (Akiskal et al., 1980; Rosenthal et al., 1981) sought to define a core group of dysthymics that responded to pharmacotherapy as defined by the pharmacological dissection strategy (Klein, 1974). Our findings led to the hypothesis that these patients could be divided into predominantly "affective" or "character spectrum" subgroups, based on their response to an adequate pharmacological trial (at least two secondary amine TCAs, lithium carbonate, or both) provided in the context of brief "practical" psychotherapy that addressed these patients' social interactional problems. Patients who responded to pharmacotherapy had the shortened REM latency (less than

70 minutes on consecutive nights) characteristic of acute primary major depression (Kupfer, 1976), but unlike classical unipolar depression, they exhibited hypersomnia. Family history was positive for both unipolar and bipolar affective disorder. The temperamental profile in many of these patients conformed to Schneider's (1958) depressive type. Although most such patients pursued a predominantly subunipolar course, about a third of them displayed subtle tendencies, as evidenced by brief hypomanic switches, on TCA challenge. Such findings suggest that in some patients, dysthymia is on a nosological continuum with cyclothymic and bipolar II disorders. Indeed, prospective studies of dysthymic children have shown bipolar switches during puberty or adolescence (Kovacs et al., 1994). This means that the predominantly unipolar course of dysthymia observed in adult psychiatric practice is in part artifactual; those dysthymics that have become bipolar during their juvenile phase, would no longer be represented in dysthymic clinical samples. Indeed, dysthymia can be detected in the prepubertal and adolescent offspring and siblings of patients with bipolar disorder (Akiskal et al., 1985). Hence, lithium or lithium augmentation is potentially useful with dysthymic patients who have a bipolar familial background (Rosenthal et al., 1981; Akiskal, 1983). This is analogous to lithium augmentation in those few major depressions—with soft bipolarity—which prove resistant to TCA monotherapy.

Sixty percent of our dysthymics failed to respond to the tricyclic agents and/or lithium carbonate as described earlier. These patients exhibited a character spectrum of dependent, histrionic, and related traits. Their REM latencies were in the normal range (70–110 minutes). Other characteristics included polydrug and alcohol abuse and high rates of familial alcoholism. These patients overlap considerably with those suffering from what Winokur (1979) called "depression spectrum disease," an early onset disorder characterized by a tempestuous life history and superimposed depressive conditions occurring in the offspring of adult alcoholic and sociopathic probands.

To date, four groups of investigators, who have used research strategies similar to those in the Tennessee studies, have published findings that support the proposed distinction between subaffective dysthymia and character spectrum disorder. For example, Hauri and Sateia (1984) confirmed our REM findings in dysthymics presenting to a sleep disorder center. Likewise, a Hungarian study by Rihmer (1990) reported positive, even hypomanic, responses to thymoleptic agents and/or sleep deprivation in inpatient dysthymics. Klein and colleagues (1988) have shown that familial bipolar illness and hypomania during prospective follow-up characterize a subgroup of early onset outpatient dysthymics. Finally, the work of Ravindran et al. (1994) represents yet another replication in delineating a pharmacotherapy-responsive subgroup within the heterogeneous universe of dysthymias (see Ravindran & Lapierre, Chapter 3, this volume).

Judging from the treatment response rate in our study (Akiskal et al., 1980), the TCA-responsive dysthymia may account for approximately 40–50% of a broadly defined chronically depressed population in community mental health centers. The Kocsis et al. report (1988), which used imipramine in a double-blind paradigm, suggests such dysthymia to be much more prevalent in outpatient private practice, possibly accounting for two-thirds of all cases of chronic depression. As newer psychopharmacological agents become available, the universe of character spectrum patients will probably shrink further. For instance, the MAOI phenelzine has been found useful in some dysthymic patients (Vallejo et al., 1987). Given such response to an MAOI, it is of interest that in the Memphis study, TCA-nonresponsive patients were of a dependent–histrionic personality type; dysthymia with such features is reminiscent of the MAOI-responsive hysteroid dysphoric patients (Liebowitz & Klein, 1979). Other agents effective in dysthymia include moclobemide (Stabl et al., 1989; Versiani et al., in press), ritanserin (Bakish et al., 1993), fluoxetine (Hellerstein et al., 1993), amisulpride (Boyer & Lecrubier, 1996), and sertraline (Thase et al., 1996).[1] A multicenter trial of paroxetine is completed but remains unpublished.

Long-Term Management of Dysthymia

The foregoing studies have demonstrated efficacy in the acute (6 weeks to 3 months) treatment of dysthymia. Clinically, it is apparent that such patients require long-term treatment. Compliance is often problematic in these patients, especially with TCAs, which produce troublesome side effects. Given the generally better tolerance profile of the SSRIs, in 1988, in collaboration with Dr. Radwan Haykal, we undertook a prospective long-term systematic open study in dysthymia with fluoxetine, the first available SSRI in the United States. The short-term results of this study (at 2-year follow-up) were presented in Washington in May 1992 at the American Psychiatric Association annual meeting. A brief report has appeared in French (Akiskal, 1993). I summarize here the methodology of that study and highlight selected findings.

The study was conducted on private outpatients, with strictly diagnosed core group of primary dysthymics based on DSM-III-R criteria. Superimposed major depression was permitted, provided prior dysthymic baseline for at least 5 years constituted patients' habitual self; concomitant panic, social phobic, and bulimic features, as well as substance abuse, were permitted as long as they did not dominate the clinical picture. The design was one of naturalistic open study, with doctor's choice treatment, with medication dose as tolerated, and psychotherapy as deemed appropriate. "Responders" were defined as unequivocal clinical recovery with DSM-III-R Axis V or general adaptive functioning (GAF) score over 70, sustained for at least 6 months. Despite long periods of prior treatment, dysthymics who entered the present study were moderately to seriously impaired in their social functioning, with DSM-III-R GAF scores in the 40s and 50s. Average prospective follow-up on fluoxetine was 2 years, dosage ranging from 20 mg every other day to 40 mg/day.

In one-third of TCA-treated patients, pharmacotherapy had to be discontinued because of intolerable side effects; the comparative figure for fluoxetine was 12%. Furthermore, the side effect profile was distinct with the two classes of antidepressants: with TCAs, it concerned the classical anticholinergic effects, weight gain and electrocardiographic changes; with fluoxetine, the reason for discontinuation was agitation.

Two-thirds of the fluoxetine group responded with a GAF above 70; half of TCA-treated dysthymics responded by this criterion. (Thyroid augmentation was used in few cases in both groups.) Patients whose lives had been immersed in lifelong gloom were rendered essentially depression-free, their functioning having been boosted by at least 20 GAF points. More remarkably, slightly more than half of all fluoxetine-responding patients—as compared to none in the TCA group—achieved even superior levels of social adaptation in the 81–90 GAF range. In DSM-III-R terms, these fluoxetine-treated patients exhibited "good functioning in all areas, interested and involved in a wide range of activities, socially effective, generally satisfied with life, no more than everyday problems or concerns." Many stated that they experienced *joie de vivre* for the first time in their lives. This group of fluoxetine-responsive patients characterized their response as "feeling comfortable to face life stresses," "no longer being overwhelmed by daily hassles," and "coping effortlessly." By contrast, 5 (of the total sample of 42 patients) who made dramatic statements such as "I feel like having a new mind," or " I am now on a higher plane of existence than anytime in my life" ultimately did poorly and seemed to have switched into bipolarity (indeed, 4 of 5 such patients had bipolar family history).

The foregoing findings suggest that an SSRI—such as fluoxetine— can considerably attenuate long-term "character" traits of poor coping, low self-esteem dependence, and resignation that were *secondary*, having resulted from the chronic dysthymic state. By contrast, the brief switch into an upper mode (hyperthymic) temperament represents action on an underlying bipolar *diathesis* rather than a genuine character change. Based on our clinical experience, patients with such switching would benefit from reduction of SSRI dose, and/or lithium, or even divalproex augmentation.

Psychotherapeutic Considerations

Factors in Treatment Failure

Any discussion of chronic depression must necessarily address the issue of treatment adequacy. Despite significant therapeutic advances, recent data (Keller et al., 1986) indicate that two out of three patients with depression, including those seen in academic psychiatric settings, do not receive adequate treatment. Inadequate treatment can result from pharmacological, patient, and physician factors (Akiskal, 1985).

Pharmacological factors include inadequate dosage or duration of antidepressant trials (which need a 3-month minimum with the SSRIs); polypharmacy with little scientific rationale; and disabling side effects, especially sexual, that result in premature interruption of treatment.

Patient factors stem from noncompliance with treatment for a variety of reasons, including rejection of a pharmacological "crutch"; a feeling of unworthiness to be helped; fear of dependence or addiction; hypochondriacal concern about side effects; and, sometimes, frank delusions of being poisoned. Other patients mistakenly interpret the prescription of antidepressants as a sign that their doctors do not care about them, that they have no interest to listen to their woes. Finally, some patients reject medication because acceptance would mean that they are as sick as a family member who committed suicide.

Certain physician attitudes may also seriously undermine treatment. A clinician who is ambivalent about using medication for a "psychological" disorder may unduly emphasize character pathology while paying minimal attention to the affective nature of the illness. A therapist, frustrated by the patient's failure to respond may, actually, find comfort in a characterological diagnosis, based on the unfounded belief that those with such diagnoses do not suffer (Price, 1978). The borderline label is especially problematic when applied to patients with tempestuous histories and unfathomable mood swings (Akiskal, 1981). It may serve as an "explanation" for a patient's poor response and thus could sabotage potentially useful somatic interventions. Other clinicians may compromise treatment compliance by failing to educate patients and their families about our current understanding of depressive illness and its treatment. Finally, physicians who rely heavily on conventional agents tend to underuse MAOIs; the logic of such reticence is the unreliability of character-disordered patients to adhere to the requisite dietary restrictions. The clinical availability of new classes of reversible MAOIs (or RIMAs) in Europe,

Canada, Mexico, and South America, would conceivably change such attitudes. Serotonergic antidepressants, which seem to possess a clinical spectrum of activity that in part overlaps with that of MAOIs, already seem to have had a positive impact on clinicians' willingness to consider pharmacotherapy for nonclassical depressions. For many patients the SSRIs have been "miraculous" in attenuating pathological postdepressive personality traits; many dysthymics feel liberated from their long-standing depressive inertia and experience the joy of a new mental and physical well-being. These and associated positive changes in coping behavior have been correlated with amelioration of serotonergic indices (Ravindran et al., 1995).

To recapitulate, multiple factors seem to underlie treatment failure for what is the most treatable of all psychiatric disorders. Many affectively ill patients are prematurely categorized as "treatment-resistant" or, worse, "characterological"—labels that can sentence the patient to long-term suffering. However, inadequate treatment or treatment resistance does not account for all cases of chronic depression; many dysthymic individuals come to clinical settings with established chronicity that predates any treatment effort.

Postdepressive Personality Changes

Interpersonal disturbances are common in patients with established chronicity of dysthymia over a decade or longer. Such disturbances are secondary to the distortions produced by long-standing depression. Observed pathological characterological changes go beyond those discussed previously and may include clinging or hostile dependence, demandingness, touchiness, pessimism, and helplessness. A dangerous stereotype exists in our field: because a patient has not responded adequately to standard treatments, because the illness has become chronic, there must be a characterological substrate to the illness. Even patients may begin to internalize such stereotypes. Thus, the long duration of the illness can lead to the patient's identification with the failing functions of depression, producing the self-image of being a "depressive person." This self-image itself represents a malignant cognitive manifestation of the depressive illness and a postdepressive personality change (Cassano et al., 1983).

For many chronic depressives, the depression is part of the fabric of their daily existence, and they might not seek help unless intensification of the illness reduces them to the level of a totally malfunctioning individual at home, at school, or in work. Others, with perhaps greater insight, might seek help at an earlier stage: They present as "existential depressions," feeling empty and without *joie de vivre* outside their work. In Germany, such individuals have been described as leading a "monocategorical existence."

This description in part reflects the shrinking of opportunities in life imposed by depression; they also reflect work as a compensatory defense against depressive disorganization (Tellenbach, 1980).

Psychological principles in the management of dysthymic patients should capitalize on the clinical observation that such individuals seem to derive personal gratification from overdedication to professions that require great service to and suffering on behalf of other people. Therefore, such patients need vocational guidance that takes the natural tendencies of their temperament into consideration (Kretschmer, 1936). Social skills training can benefit dysthymics whose life has been paralyzed because of introversion; it must be borne in mind, however, that psychological approaches alone often fail in the absence of competent pharmacotherapy, which is necessary to reverse the depressive inertia and joylessness so characteristic of the somber life of many dysthymic patients (Akiskal et al., 1980; Friedman et al., 1995).

Supportive and Psychoeducational Approaches

The long-term psychopharmacological management of this very complex group of chronic patients is still very much of an art that each clinician must develop by informed "trial and error" on a large number of patients examined over long periods of personal follow-up. Such experience teaches the physician that psychoeducation and psychotherapeutic approaches can considerably enhance the gains made through chemotherapy.

However, long-term psychotherapy deriving from psychodynamic theory, commonly used with the ambition to modify the character pathology in depressives (Arieti & Bemporad, 1978), is of unproven value for this purpose. To put it bluntly, personality disturbances observed in chronic affective conditions represent constitutional givens which are minimally responsive to insight-oriented therapies, or epiphenomenal to the affective pathology and unlikely to recede without significant improvement in this pathology. More focused practical supportive and interpersonal interventions (Weissman & Akiskal, 1984; Markowitz, 1994) and psychoeducational approaches for both patient and spouse are needed to combat the demoralization of a chronic illness with devastating effects on scholastic, vocational, and personal life and to enhance rapport, hope, and compliance with medication regimens (Akiskal, 1992b). Most important, the treating clinician should maintain an attitude of optimism and inform the patient of the increasing availability of more specific thymoleptic agents. Maintaining empathy is not always easy, as many chronic depressives tend to irritate and alienate their doctors. In the case of these more impulsive, dysphoric patients, it is necessary to set clear limits right from the outset of treatment:

Repeated angry outbursts directed at the physician are countertherapeutic and will not be tolerated, as they signal the destructive effect of anger on interpersonal relationships outside therapy.

We have already noted how mediocre responses to halfhearted attempts to treat chronic depression might lead the clinician to change the patient's diagnosis to character disorder. Affective reconceptualization of "character" disorders within a biological framework not only brings the potential benefit of innovative psychopharmacological strategies to this "difficult" group of patients but could reduce physicians' countertransference to the patient and thereby lead to more efficient treatment.

The long-term clinical care of patients with chronic affective dysregulation requires versatility in biological and psychosocial interventions as well as the stamina to endure their hopeless despair which is often "contagious," especially when treatment is not progressing at all. Treating clinicians themselves may need periodic support; indeed, such patients are best treated in the setting of group practice.

Pulling out of despair patients "written off" as incurable by themselves, their family, or previous therapists is one of the most gratifying professional experiences in the field of medicine. Despite opinion to the contrary, depressives with personality disorders do respond to antidepressants (Downs et al., 1992). Even malignant characterological distortions brought about by protracted depression can often be attenuated (Akiskal, 1992b) with the sophisticated psychopharmacological care available today for chronic affective conditions.

Vocational guidance that attempts to match the patient's temperament to a specific type of work or object choice in which he or she will be in optimum harmony ultimately represents a more realistic goal than modifying the personality structure (Akiskal & Akiskal, 1992). For instance, those patients who are unable to get up at the "societal" hours of 6 to 7 A.M. to go to work should be encouraged to seek jobs with more flexible hours; only a minority do benefit from terminal sleep deprivation.

Conclusion

What emerges from this review is the heterogeneity of the large terrain of ambulatory, low-grade, protracted depressive symptomatology. Despite considerable overlap with personality disorders from the "anxious" and to some extent "dramatic" clusters, I have attempted to illustrate the heuristic value of considering them as variants of affective disorders. The rationale for such reconceptualization can now be defended by external validation strategies such as course of illness, family history, biological markers, and pharmacological dissection (Akiskal, 1983; Howland & Thase, 1991; Akiskal, 1996). Such data are strongest for dysthymia (Table 1.4). North American clinicians have generally responded with increased enthusiasm for the use of pharmacological interventions in chronic affective conditions with characterological taint (Shader et al., 1990). Even psychoanalytically oriented psychiatrists now tend to endorse the view that in special chronic depressive subgroups the character pathology represents a defense against an underlying affective dysregulation (Cooper, 1985).

Contrary to clinical lore, many personality attributes intimately related to the affective pathology improve significantly with competent pharmacotherapy that uses the appropriate dosage and duration (Kocsis et al., 1988; Rouillon et al., 1989; Stewart et al., 1988; Downs et al., 1992). Physicians should therefore attempt vigorous pharmacological interventions in most forms of chronic depression; with continued pharmacotherapy, beneficial effects can be maintained much beyond the index phase for which the patient sought help (Akiskal, 1993; Kocsis et al., 1996). Although concurrent psychotherapeutic interventions can enhance the gains made by pharmacotherapy, psychotherapy alone proves inadequate for many of these patients (Akiskal et al., 1989). This is not to say that all characterological disturbances will melt away in response to chemotherapy, but it is to suggest that such pathology does not bar dysthymia from significant response to thymoleptic agents.

Finally, the various treatments outlined—whether psychological or biological—should aim primarily to reduce disabling symptoms and behaviors; basic temperamental traits are least likely to change, and therapists must endeavor to gently steer dysthymic individuals toward educational experiences, vocational experiences, and object choices most suited to their natural–constitutional inclinations. In closing, it is appropriate to remind the reader of Schneider's (1958) admonition that work is the best therapy for individuals with depressive personality attributes. Such individuals feel their greatest harmony in work. When such harmony is achieved, medication dosage can be reduced gradually and, in selected cases, eliminated

TABLE 1.4. Evidence for Considering Dysthymia as a Subaffective Disorder

Familial affective loading (unipolar and bipolar)
Diurnality of inertia, gloom, and anhedonia
Phase advance of REM sleep
TRH–TSH Challenge Test abnormalities
Prospective course complicated by major affective episodes
Response to sleep deprivation
Response to selected thymoleptics
Spontaneous or pharmacological hypomania

Note. Data from Akiskal (1994a).

altogether. Any potential benefits from more formal psychotherapy must await controlled trials (Markowitz, 1994).

Acknowledgment

Radwan Haykal, MD, Charter Lakeside Mood Disorders Program, Memphis, took part in several of the studies reviewed in this chapter.

Note

1. Moclobemide, ritanserin, and amisulpride are not marketed in the United States. In the author's experience, trifluoperazine 1 mg/day acts like the dopaminergic amisulpride and is sometimes efficacious in resistant dysthymics (especially those with bipolar family history).

References

Akiskal, H. S. (1981). Subaffective disorders: Dysthymic, cyclothymic and bipolar II disorders in the "borderline" realm. *Psychiatric Clinics of North America, 4,* 25-46.

Akiskal, H. S. (1982). Factors associated with incomplete recovery in primary depressive illness. *Journal of Clinical Psychiatry, 43,* 266-271.

Akiskal, H. S. (1983). Dysthymic disorder: Psychopathology of proposed chronic depressive subtypes. *American Journal of Psychiatry, 140,* 11-20.

Akiskal, H. S. (1984). Characterologic manifestations of affective disorders: Toward a new conceptualization. *Integrative Psychiatry, 2,* 83-96.

Akiskal, H. S. (1985). A proposed clinical approach to chronic and "resistant" depressions: Evaluation and treatment. *Journal of Clinical Psychiatry, 46,* 32-37.

Akiskal, H. S. (1986) A developmental perspective on recurrent mood disorders: A review of studies in man. *Psychopharmacology Bulletin, 22,* 579-586.

Akiskal, H. S. (1990a). Toward a clinical understanding of the relationship of anxiety and depressive disorders. In J. Maser & R. Cloninger (Eds.), *Comorbidity in anxiety and mood disorders* (pp. 597-607). Washington, DC: American Psychiatric Press.

Akiskal, H. S. (1990b). Toward a definition of dysthymia: Boundaries with personality and mood disorders. In S. W. Burton & H. S. Akiskal (Eds.), *Dysthymic disorder* (pp. 1-12). London: Gaskell.

Akiskal, H. S. (1991). Chronic depression. *Bulletin of the Menninger Clinic, 55,* 156-171.

Akiskal, H. S. (1992a). Le déprime avant la dépression [The depression before the depression]. *L'Encephale, 18,* 485-489.

Akiskal, H. S. (1992b). Psychopharmacologic and psychotherapeutic strategies in intermittent and chronic affective conditions. In S. A. Montgomery & F. Rouillon (Eds.), *Long-term treatment of depression* (pp. 43–62). Chichester, UK: Wiley.

Akiskal, H. S. (1993). La dysthymie et son traitement. *L'Encephale, 19,* 375–378.

Akiskal, H. S. (1994a). Dysthymic and cyclothymic depressions: Therapeutic implications. *Journal of Clinical Psychiatry, 55*(Suppl. 4), 46–52.

Akiskal, H. S. (1994b). The temperamental borders of affective disorders. *Acta Psychiatrica Scandinavica, 379*(Suppl.), 32–37.

Akiskal, H. S. (1996). Dysthymia as a temperamental variant of affective disorder. *European Psychiatry, 11*(Suppl. 3), 117s–122s.

Akiskal, H. S., & Akiskal, K. (1992). Cyclothymic, hyperthymic and depressive temperaments as subaffective variants of mood disorders. In A. Tasman & M. B. Riba (Eds.), *American Psychiatric Association review* (pp. 43–62). Washington, DC: American Psychiatric Press.

Akiskal, H. S., Bitar, A. H., Puzantian, V. R., Rosenthal, T. L., & Walker, P. W. (1978). The nosological status of neurotic depression: A prospective three- to four-year follow-up examination in light of the primary–secondary and unipolar–bipolar dichotomies. *Archives of General Psychiatry, 35,* 756–766.

Akiskal, H. S., Downs, J. M., Jordan, P., Watson, S., Daugherty, D., & Pruitt, D. B. (1985). Affective disorders in referred children and younger siblings of manic–depressives. *Archives of General Psychiatry, 42,* 996–1003.

Akiskal, H. S., Haykal, F. R., & Downs, J. M. (1989). Overview of chronic-resistant depressions. *Psychiatry in the 80's, 7,* 1–3.

Akiskal, H. S., & Lemmi, H. (1987). Sleep EEG findings bearing on the relationship of anxiety and depressive disorders. In G. Recagani & E. Smeraldi (Eds.), *Anxious depression: Assessment and treatment* (pp. 153–159). New York: Raven Press.

Akiskal, H. S., & Mallya, G. (1987). Criteria for the "soft" bipolar spectrum: Treatment implications. *Psychopharmacology Bulletin, 23,* 68–73.

Akiskal, H. S., Rosenthal, T. L., Haykal, R. F., Lemmi, H., Rosenthal, R. H., & Scott-Strauss, A. (1980). Characterologic depressions: Clinical and sleep EEG findings separating "subaffective dysthymias" from "character spectrum disorders." *Archives of General Psychiatry, 37,* 777–783.

Akiskal, H. S., Walker, P., Puzantian, V. R., King, D., Rosenthal, T. L., & Dranon, M. (1983). Bipolar outcome in the course of depressive illness: Phenomenologic, familial, and pharmacologic predictors. *Journal of Affective Disorders, 5,* 115–128.

Akiskal, H. S., & Weise, R. E. (1992). The clinical spectrum of so-called "minor" depression. *American Journal of Psychotherapy, 46,* 9–22.

American Psychiatric Association. (1980). *Diagnostic and statistical manual of mental disorders* (3rd ed.). Washington, DC: Author.

American Psychiatric Association. (1987). *Diagnostic and statistical manual of mental disorders* (3rd ed., rev.). Washington, DC: Author.

American Psychiatric Association. (1994). *Diagnostic and statistical manual of mental disorders* (4th ed.). Washington, DC: Author.

Andrews, G., Stewart, G., Morris-Yates, A., Holt, P., & Henderson, S. (1990). Evidence for a general neurotic syndrome. *British Journal of Psychiatry, 157*, 6–12.

Angst, J. (1992). Comorbidity of recurrent brief depression. *Clinical Neuropharmacology, 15*, 9A–10A.

Angst, J., Merikangas, K., Scheidegger, P., & Wicki, W. (1990). Recurrent brief depression: A new subtype of affective disorder. *Journal of Affective Disorders, 19*, 87–98.

Arieti, S., & Bemporad, J. (1978). *Severe and mild depression.* New York: Basic Books.

Bakish, D., Lapierre, Y. D., Weinstein, R., Klein, J., Wiens, A., Jones, B., Horn, E., Browne, M., Bourget, D., Blanchard, A., et al. (1993). Ritanserin, imipramine, and placebo in the treatment of dysthymic disorder. *Journal of Clinical Psychopharmacology, 13*, 409–414.

Beard, G. M. (1881). *A practical treatise on nervous exhaustion (neurasthenia): Its nature, sequences, and treatment.* New York: W. Wood.

Bonime, W. (1966). The psychodynamics of neurotic depression. In S. Arieti (Ed.), *American handbook of psychiatry* (Vol. 1, pp. 239–255). New York: Basic Books.

Boyer, P., & Lecrubier, Y. (1996). Atypical antipsychotic drugs in dysthymia: Placebo controlled studies of amisulpride versus imipramine, versus amineptine. *European Psychiatry, 11*(Suppl. 3), 135s–140s.

Bronisch, T., Wittchen, H. U., Krieg, C., Rupp, H. U., & von Zerssen, D. (1985). Depressive neurosis: A long-term prospective and retrospective follow-up study of former in-patients. *Acta Psychiatrica Scandinavica, 71*, 237–248.

Burton, S. W., & Akiskal, H. S. (Eds.). (1990). *Dysthymic disorder.* London: Gaskell.

Cassano, G. B., Akiskal, H. S., Perugi, G., Musetti, L., & Savino, M. (1992). The importance of measures of affective temperaments in genetic studies of mood disorders. *Journal of Psychiatric Research, 26*, 257–268.

Cassano, G. B., Maggini, C., & Akiskal, H. S. (1983). Short-term, subchronic, and chronic sequelae of afective disorders. *Psychiatric Clinics of North America, 6*, 55–67.

Chodoff, P. (1972). The depressive personality: A critical review. *Archives of General Psychiatry, 27*, 666–673.

Clayton, P. J., Grove, W. M., Coryell, W., Keller, M., Hirschfeld, R., & Fawcett, J. (1991). Follow-up and family study of anxious depression. *American Journal of Psychiatry, 148*(11), 1512–1517.

Cooper, A. M. (1985). Will neurology influence psychoanalysis? *American Journal of Psychiatry, 142*, 1395–1402.

Coryell, W., Endicott, J., & Keller, M. (1992). Anxiety syndromes as epiphenomena of primary major depression: Outcome and familial psychopathology. *American Journal of Psychiatry, 149*(1), 100–107.

Davidson, J. R., Miller, R. D., Turnbull, C. D., & Sullivan, J. L. (1982). Atypical depression. *Archives of General Psychiatry, 39*, 527–534.

de Montigny, C., Grunberg, F., Mayer, A., & Deschenes, J. P. (1981). Lithium induces rapid relief of depression in TCA drug non-responders. *British Journal of Psychiatry, 138*, 252–256.

Downs, N. S., Swerdlow, N. R., & Zisook, S. (1992). The relationship of affective illness and personality disorders in psychiatric outpatients. *Annals of Clinical Psychiatry, 4,* 87–94.

Ebert, D., & Barocka, A. (1991). The early course of atypical depression. *European Archives of Psychiatry and Clinical Neuroscience, 241,* 131–132.

Freidman, R. A., Markowitz, J. C., Parides, M., & Kocsis, J. H. (1995). Acute response of social functioning in dysthymic patients with desipramine. *Journal of Affective Disorders, 34*(2), 85–88.

Gershon, E. S., Hamovit, J., Guroff, J. J., Dibble, E., Leckman, J. F., Sceery, W., Targum, S. D., Nurnberger, J. I., Jr., Goldin, L. R., & Bunney, W. E., Jr. (1982). A family study of schizoaffective, bipolar I, bipolar II, unipolar, and normal control probands. *Archives of General Psychiatry, 39,* 1157–1167.

Goodwin, D. W., Schulsinger, F., Knop, J., Mednick, S., & Guze, S. B. (1977). Psychopathology in adopted and nonadopted daughters of alcoholics. *Archives of General Psychiatry, 34,* 1005–1009.

Greenberg, D. B. (1990). Neurasthenia in the 1980's: Chronic mononucleosis, chronic fatigue syndrome, and anxiety and depressive disorders. *Psychosomatics, 31,* 129–137.

Hauri, P., & Sateia, M. J. (1984). REM sleep in dysthymic disorders. *Sleep Research, 13,* 119.

Hellerstein, D. J., Yanowitch, P., Rosenthal, J., Samstag, L. W., Maurer, M., Kasch, K., Burrows, L., Poster, M., Cantillon, M., & Winston, A. (1993). A randomized double-blind study of fluoxetine versus placebo in the treatment of dysthymia. *American Journal of Psychiatry, 150,* 1169–1175.

Himmelhoch, J. M., Thase, M. E., Mallinger, A. G., & Houck, P. (1991). Tranylcypromine versus imipramine in anergic bipolar depression. *American Journal of Psychiatry, 148,* 910–916.

Hirschfeld, R. M. A., Klerman, G. L., Lavori, P., Keller, M. B., Griffith, P., & Coryell, W. (1989). Premorbid personality assessments of first onset of major depression. *Archives of General Psychiatry, 46,* 345–350.

Howland, R. H. (1991). Pharmacotherapy of dysthymia: A review. *Journal of Clinical Psychopharmacology, 11,* 83–92.

Jaspers, K. (1962). *General psychopathology* (J. Hoenig & M. H. Hamilton, Trans.). Manchester: Manchester University Press.

Judd, L. L., Rapaport, M. H., Paulus, M. P., & Brown, J. L. (1994). Subsyndromal symptomatic depression: A new mood disorder? *Journal of Clinical Psychiatry, 55*(Suppl. 4), 18–28.

Kasahara, Y. (1991). The practical diagnosis of depression in Japan. In J. P. Feighner & W. F. Boyer (Eds.), *The diagnosis of depression* (pp. 163–175). Chichester: Wiley.

Keller, M. B. (1994). Course, outcome and impact on the community. *Acta Psychiatrica Scandinavica, 89*(Suppl. 383), 24–34.

Keller, M. B., Lavori, P. W., Andreason, N. C., Endicott, J., Coryell, W., Fawcett, J., Rice, J. P., & Hirschfeld, R. M. (1986). Low levels and lack of predictors of somatotherapy and psychotherapy received by depressed patients. *Archives of General Psychiatry, 43,* 458–466.

Keller, M. B., Lavori, P. W., Endicott, J., Coryell, W., & Klerman, G. L. (1983). "Double depression": Two year follow-up. *American Journal of Psychiatry, 140,* 689–694.

Kendall, P. C., & Watson, D. (1989). *Anxiety and depression: Distinctive and overlapping features.* San Diego: Academic Press.

Kendler, K. S., Neale, M. C., Kessler, R. C., Heath, A. C., & Eaves, L. J. (1992). Major depression and generalized anxiety disorder. Same genes (partly) different environments. *Archives of General Psychiatry, 49,* 716–722.

Kernberg, O. F. (1986). A psychoanalytic classification of character pathology. In *Object-relations theory and clinical psychoanalysis.* Northvale, NJ: Jason Aronson.

Klein, D. F. (1974). Endogenomorphic depression: A conceptual and terminological revision. *Archives of General Psychiatry, 31,* 447–454.

Klein, D. N. (1990). Depressive personality. *Journal of Abnormal Psychology, 99,* 412–421.

Klein, D. N., Taylor, E. B., Harding, K., & Dickstein, S. (1988). Double depression and episodic major depression: Demographic, clinical, familial, personality, and socioenvironmental characteristics and short-term outcome. *American Journal of Psychiatry, 145,* 1226–1231.

Kleinman, A. (1986). *Social origins of distress and disease: Depression, neurasthenia, and pain in modern China.* New Haven: Yale University Press.

Klerman, G. L., Endicott, J., Spitzer, R., & Hirschfeld, R. M. (1979). Neurotic depressions: A systematic analysis of multiple criteria and meanings. *American Journal of Psychiatry, 136,* 57–61.

Kocsis, J. H., Frances, A. J., Voss, C., Mann, J. J., Mason, B. J., & Sweeney, J. (1988). Imipramine treatment for chronic depression. *Archives of General Psychiatry, 45,* 253–257.

Kocsis, J. H., Friedman, R. A., Markowitz, J. C., Leon, A. C., Miller, N. L., Gniwesch, L., & Parides, M. (1996). Maintenance therapy for chronic depression. *Archives of General Psychiatry, 53,* 769–774.

Koukopoulos, A., Reginaldi, D., Laddomada, P., Floris, G., Serra, G., & Tondo, L. (1980). Course of the manic–depressive cycle and changes caused by treatment. *Pharmacopsychiatric Neuropsychopharmcology, 13,* 156–167.

Kovacs, M., Akiskal, H. S., Gatsonis, C., & Parrone, P. L. (1994). Childhood-onset dysthymic disorder: Clinical features and prospective naturalistic outcome. *Archives of General Psychiatry, 51,* 365–374.

Kraepelin, E. (1921). *Manic–depressive insanity and paranoia* (R. M. Barclay, Trans.; G. M. Robertson, Ed.). Edinburgh: E. S. Livingstone.

Kraines, S. H. (1957). *Mental depressions and their treatment.* New York: Macmillan.

Kretschmer, E. (1936). *Physique and character* (E. Miller, Trans.). London: Kegan, Paul.

Kupfer, D. J. (1976). REM latency: A psychobiological marker for primary depressive disease. *Biological Psychiatry, 11,* 159–174.

Liebowitz, M. R., & Klein, D. F. (1979). Hysteroid dysphoria. *Psychiatric Clinics of North America, 2,* 555–575.

Liebowitz, M. R., Quitkin, F. M., Stewart, J. W., McGrath, P. J., Harrison, W. M., Markowitz, J. S., Rabkin, J. G., Tricamo, E., Goetz, D. M., & Klein, D. F. (1988).

Antidepressant specificity in atypical depression: A family study perspective. *Journal of Affective Disorders, 24,* 129–137.

Maier, W., Lichtermann, D., Minges, J., & Heun, R. (1992). Personality traits in subjects at risk for unipolar major depression: A family study perspective. *Journal of Affective Disorders, 24,* 153–163.

Markowitz, J. C. (1994). Psychotherapy of dysthymia. *American Journal of Psychiatry, 151,* 1114–1121.

Markowitz, J. C., Moran, M. E., Kocsis, J. H., & Frances, A. J. (1992). Prevalence and comorbidity of dysthymic disorder among psychiatric outpatients. *Journal of Affective Disorders, 24,* 63–71.

Maser, J. D., & Cloninger, C. R. (Eds.). (1990). *Comorbidity of mood and anxiety disorders.* Washington, DC: American Psychiatric Press.

Montgomery, S. A., Montgomery, D., Baldwin, D., & Green, M. (1989). Intermittent 3-day depressions and suicidal behavior. *Neuropsychopharmacology, 22,* 128–134.

Mueller, T., Lavori, P., Keller, M., Swartz, A., Warshaw, M., Hasin, D., Coryell, W., Endicott, J., Rice, J., & Akiskal H. S. (1994). The prognostic effect of the variable course of alcoholism on the ten-year course of depression. *American Journal of Psychiatry, 151,* 199–204.

Musetti, L., Perugi, G., Soriani, A., Rossi, V. M., Cassano, G. B., & Akiskal H. S. (1989). Depression before and after age 65: A re-examination. *British Journal of Psychiatry, 155,* 330–336.

Parker, G., Blignault, I., & Manicavasagar, V. (1988). Neurotic depression: Delineation of symptom profiles and their relation to outcome. *British Journal of Psychiatry, 152,* 15–23.

Paskind, H. A. (1929). Brief attacks of manic–depressive depression. *Archives of Neurological Psychiatry, 22,* 123–134.

Peron-Magnan, P. (1992). Trouble dysthymique et personnalité dépressive. *L'Encephale, 18,* 51–54.

Perugi, G., Akiskal, H. S., Musetti, L., Simonini, E., & Cassano, G. B. (1994). Social adjustment in panic-agoraphobic patients reconsidered. *British Journal of Psychiatry, 164,* 88–93.

Perugi, G., Musetti, L., Simonini, E., Piagentini, F., Cassano, G. B., & Akiskal H. S. (1990). Gender-mediated clinical features of depressive illness: The importance of temperamental differences. *British Journal of Psychiatry, 164,* 88–93.

Post, R. M., Uhde, T. W., & Roy-Byrne, P. P. (1986). Antidepressant effects of carbamazepine. *American Journal of Psychiatry, 43,* 29–34.

Price, J. S. (1978). Chronic depressive illness. *British Medical Journal, 1,* 1200–1201.

Ravindran, A. V., Bialik, R. J., & Lapierre, Y. D. (1994). Therapeutic efficacy of specific serotonin reuptake inhibitors (SSRIs) in dysthymia. *Canadian Journal of Psychiatry, 39,* 21–26.

Ravindran, A. V., Griffiths, J., Waddell, C., & Anisman, H. (1995). Stressful life events and coping styles in relation to dysthymia and major depressive disorder: Variations associated with alleviation of symptoms following pharmacotherapy. *Progress in Neuro-Psychopharmacology and Biological Psychiatry, 19*(4), 637–653.

Rifkin, A., Quitkin, F., Carrillo, C., Blumberg, A. G., & Klein, D. F. (1972). Lithium carbonate in emotionally unstable character disorder. *Archives of General Psychiatry, 27,* 519–523.

Rihmer, Z. (1990). Dysthymia—a clinician's perspective. In S. W. Burton & H. S. Akiskal (Eds.), *Dysthymic disorder* (pp. 112–125). London: Gaskell.

Robins, L. N., & Regier, D. A. (Eds.). (1991). *Psychiatric disorders in America.* New York: Free Press.

Rosenthal, T. L., Akiskal, H. S., Scott-Strauss, A., Rosenthal, R. H., & David, M. (1981). Familial and developmental factors in characterologic depressions. *Journal of Affective Disorders, 3,* 183–192.

Rouillon, F., Serrurier, D., Miller, H. D., & Gerard, M. J. (1991). Prophylactic efficacy of maprotiline on unipolar depression relapse. *Journal of Clinical Psychiatry, 52,* 423–431.

Sargent, W. (1962). The treatment of anxiety status and atypical depressions by the monoamine oxidase inhibitor drugs. *Journal of Neuropsychiatry, 3,* 96–103.

Savino, M., Perugi, G., Simonini, E., Soriani, A., Cassano, G. B., & Akiskal, H. S. (1993). Affective comorbidity in panic disorder: Is there a bipolar connection? *Journal of Affective Disorders, 28,* 155–163.

Schneider, K. (1958). *Psychopathic personalities* (M. W. Hamilton, Trans.). Springfield, IL: Charles C. Thomas.

Scott, J. (1988). Chronic depression. *British Journal of Psychiatry, 153,* 287–297.

Shader, R. I., Scharfman, E. L., & Dreyfuss, D. A. (1985). Toward a psychobiologic view of selected personality disorders. *Psychiatry, 1,* 1–11.

Simons, R. C. (1987). Psychoanalytic contributors to psychiatric nosology: Forms of masochistic behavior. *Journal of American Psychoanalytic Association, 35,* 583–608.

Stabl, M., Biziere, K., Schmid-Burgk, W., & Amrein, R. (1989). Review of comparative clinical trials. Moclobemide vs. TCAs and vs. placebo in depressive states. *Journal of Neural Transmitters, 28*(Suppl.), 77–89.

Stewart, J. W., Quitkin, F. M., McGrath, P. J., Rabkin, J. G., Markowitz, J. S., Tricamo, E., & Klein, D. F. (1988). Social functioning in chronic depression: effect of 6 weeks of antidepressant treatment. *Psychiatry Research, 25,* 213–222.

Tellenbach, H. (1980). *Melancholia* (E. Eng, Trans.). Pittsburgh: Dusquesne University Press.

Thase, M. E., Fava, M., Halbreich, U., Kocsis, J. H., Koran, L., Davidson, J., Rosenbaum, J., & Harrison, W. (1996). A placebo-controlled, randomized clinical trial comparing sertraline and imipramine for the treatment of dysthymia. *Archives of General Psychiatry, 53,* 777–784.

Tyrer, P., Seivewright, N., Ferguson, B., & Tyrer, J. (1992). The general neurotic syndrome: A coaxial diagnosis of anxiety, depression and personality disorder. *Acta Psychiatrica Scandinavica, 85,* 201–206.

Vallejo, J., Gasto, C., Catalan, R., & Salamero, M. (1987). Double-blind study of imipramine versus phenelzine in melancholias and dysthymic disorders. *British Journal of Psychiatry, 151,* 639–642.

Van Valkenburg, C., Akiskal, H. S., Puzantian, V., & Rosenthal, T. (1984). Anxious depressions. *Journal of Affective Disorders, 6*, 67–82.

Versiani, M., Amrein, R., & Stable, M. (in press). Moclobemide and imipramine in chronic depression (dysthymia). *Journal of International Clinical Psychopharmacology.*

von Zerssen, D. (1993). Normal and abnormal variants of premorbid personality in functional mental disorders: Conceptual and methodological themes. *Journal of Personality Disorders, 7*, 116–136.

Wehr, T. A., & Goodwin, F. K. (1987). Can antidepressants cause mania and worsen the course of affective illness? *American Journal of Psychiatry, 144*, 1403–1411.

Weissman, M. M., & Akiskal, H. S. (1984). The role of psychotherapy in chronic depressions: A proposal. *Comprehensive Psychiatry, 25*, 23–31.

Weissman, M. M., & Klerman, G. L. (1977). The chronic depressive in the community: Unrecognized and poorly tested. *Comprehensive Psychiatry, 18*, 523–532.

Wessely, S. (1990). Old wine in new bottles: Neurasthenia and "ME." *Psychology of Medicine, 20*, 35–53.

West, E. D., & Dally, P. J. (1959). Effects of iproniazid in depressive syndromes. *British Medical Journal, 1*, 1491–1494.

Widiger, T. A. (Guest Ed.). (1987). The self-defeating personality disorder. *Journal of Personality Disorders* (Special Feature), *1*, 157–201.

Winokur, G. (1979). Unipolar depression: Is it divisible into autonomous subtypes?. *Archives of General Psychiatry, 36*, 47–52.

Winokur, G. (1987). Family (genetic) studies in neurotic depression. *Journal of Psychiatric Research, 21*, 357–363.

World Health Organization. (1992). *International classification of diseases* (10th ed.). Geneva: Author.

Wolpe, J. (1988). The renascence of neurotic depression: Its varied dynamics and implications for outcome research. *Journal of Nervous Mental Disorders, 176*, 607–613.

CHAPTER 2

Dysthymia: Clinical Picture, Comorbidity, and Outcome

Marcio Versiani
A. Egidio Nardi

The purpose of this chapter is to describe the clinical features of dysthymia and its comorbidity (especially with anxiety disorders) and to discuss outcome in light of ongoing long-term treatment studies at our center.

Dysthymia in Latin America

In the course of our research program on depression during the last 8 years—and as part of a multicenter study—we recruited a sample of 276 patients suffering from dysthymia according to the DSM-III-R criteria (American Psychiatric Association, 1987). Press interviews were the main method of recruitment. We had done this before with other disorders, especially social phobia and panic disorder, and were able to gather large samples (Versiani et al., 1986, 1992). Although this method of recruiting patients is far from perfect in the sense of achieving a true community sample, it may be better for research purposes than using patients referred to clinical settings. At least in metropolitan clinical settings in Latin America, patients tend to be very severely ill, with an excess of comorbidity, extensive prior treatments, and low compliance associated with socioeconomic disorganization. In fact, in Brazilian psychiatric settings, patients with dysthymia or social phobia are rarely seen.

We used several assessment instruments to screen candidates for the dysthymia project: the Structured Clinical Interview for DSM-III-R (Spitzer et al., 1987), Hamilton Rating Scale for Depression (Hamilton, 1959), Sheehan Disabilities Scales (Sheehan, 1986), Hopkins Symptom Checklist–90 (Derogatis et al., 1973), and Social Adjustment Scale (Weissman et al., 1978). The objectives of this project were to assess the clinical presentation of the disorder, its comorbidity, the long-term outcome, responses to treatments, comparisons with other disorders—in brief, to assess whether these patients exist as described in DSM-III-R, their history, and their prognosis. Our main thrust was to include "primary dysthymia."

Demographic Characteristics

The demographic characteristics of the sample are shown in Table 2.1. These demographic characteristics agree with those of other papers in the literature (e.g., Kocsis et al. 1988). At index evaluation, the patients were predominantly female, in their 40s. The clinical characteristics are shown in Table 2.2.

We divided our patients into three groups: "pure dysthymia," "double depression at screen," and "past double depression." Here, the figures for pure dysthymia differ from reports in the literature, in which double depression appears to predominate (Kocsis et al., 1988). We suggest that this is a result of the recruitment process employed in our study (i.e., candidates were not obtained by clinical referral), which is corroborated by the fact that 66.7% of the sample never received any kind of treatment.

Comorbidity was relatively high, especially for anxiety disorders. A high prevalence of somatoform disorders was also found. Contrary to the U.S. literature (Kocsis et al., 1986; Akiskal & Weise, 1992), Axis II disorders were uncommon in our sample, which again may be explained by our selection procedure. Whatever Axis II disorders were uncovered were in Cluster C, reinforcing the link with the spectrum of anxiety disorders.

TABLE 2.1. Demographic Characteristics

Number of patients: 276
Age: mean = 40.6 years (SD = 11.5)
Sex: male 28.3%, female 71.7%
Race: white 97.8%, black 2.2%
Education: high school 57.2%, university 42.8%

Age of onset was difficult to determine. Most patients reported symptoms dating back to childhood. As Akiskal (1983) has so aptly described, these patients cannot point to a precise date of onset of their illness. Figures such as ours and those from other authors signaling mean age at onset by mid- to late adolescence may well be an artifact. What the patients may be saying is that they "became aware of the problem" by that time; most seemed to have started, insidiously, much earlier.

Comorbidity

In gathering this sample of dysthymic patients we endeavored to include primary dysthymia according to DSM-III-R. In cases of comorbidity with either social phobia or generalized anxiety disorder, this is not easy. When interviewing patients in their 40s who have had these two disorders for more than 20 years, it is difficult to determine which started first. Patients included in the study said that the gloominess they felt for as long as they remembered was their main problem. Furthermore, in cases of comorbidity with social phobia, the presentation of the latter disorder, although fulfilling the DSM-III-R criteria, is somewhat different from "pure" social phobia. The patients do fear situations in which they may be exposed to the scrutiny of others and do present anxiety symptoms in these situations (criterion A, DSM-III-R). However, their fear is subtly different from that of pure social phobics (i.e., they feel inadequate, sad, isolated, and unable to share happy experiences with others). They would prefer to stay at home, not because of a phobia but because of the "lack of pleasure of enjoying contact with others, strangers or intimate people equally."

In other comorbid cases, it was easier to determine primary dysthymia. Thus, panic disorder had a clear onset in time. The same was true for alcohol abuse or alcohol dependence. Somatoform disorders were also clearly secondary to dysthymic symptoms, at least in terms of chronology. Indeed, somatoform disorders appear to be consequences of dysthymic symptoms. However, the development of a somatoform disorder can further aggravate the dysthymia, as shown in the following vignette:

> After more than 6 years of severe dysthymic symptoms, this 21-year-old patient became excessively preoccupied with his physical appearance. He could no longer go to the beach, and avoided all girls who approached him—"they cannot like me, because I am very ugly, and my hair is wrong" and "that makes me even more sad." The dysmorphophobia here seemed to arise from a dysthymic baseline.

Relationships between dysthymia and Axis II disorders are, as expected, even more difficult to analyze. Avoidant or dependent traits (Table 2.2) are understandable in the context of the dysthymic symptom complex. The same can generally be said about obsessive–compulsive traits.

Psychopathology

We attempted to explore more thoroughly the symptomatology of our sample of 276 dysthymic patients. Of the six symptoms listed in criterion B of DSM-III-R, the main ones reported were "low energy or fatigue" (76%), "low self-esteem" (72%), "poor concentration" (65%), and "feelings of hopelessness" (64%). Contrasting what our patients reported with the list of symptoms for a major depressive episode in DSM-III-R, "observed psychomotor agitation or retardation," "inappropriate guilt," and "recurrent thoughts of death" were rare in dysthymia (less than 5%); "insomnia and hypersomnia" was present in 21%, and "poor appetite or overeating"

TABLE 2.2. Illness Characteristics and Previous Treatments

Diagnosis
  Pure dysthymia: 55.4%
  Double depression at screen: 27.5%
  Past double depression: 17.1%

Age of onset
  Mean = 16.2 years (*SD* = 7.2)

Comorbidity
  Alcohol abuse: 16.3%
  Alcohol dependence: 6.5%
  Hypochondriasis: 19.9%
  Body dysmorphic disorder: 13.0%
  Somatization disorder: 11.6%
  Axis II disorders: 16.3% (anxious cluster)
  Generalized anxiety disorder: 28.3%
  Panic disorder: 12.7%
  Social phobia: 16.3%

Previous treatments
  None: 66.7%
  Medication: 22.5%
  Psychotherapy: 19.9%
  Both: 9.1%

was present in 24% (again, considerably less than what one generally observes in major depressives).

It is also noteworthy that "thoughts of death" in dysthymic patients, at least in this sample, are rather different from those seen in typical major depression. The patients stated that sometimes they feel they would be better off dead, but they do not have plans for suicide and most, in fact, do fear death a lot. A patient described it as follows: "I don't know, sometimes I think life is not worth living, especially in the conditions I go through, but I fear death tremendously, and that is why I look for doctors."

Thus, the overlap between dysthymia and major depression with the resulting diagnosis of double depression seems to rely mainly on observed psychomotor disturbance, profound appetite or sleep disturbance, guilt, and suicidal tendencies. Problems in the overlap of dysthymia and major depression have been discussed by others (Keller & Shapiro, 1982; Akiskal, 1983; Kocsis & Frances, 1987). The data presented here may contribute to this discussion in an objective fashion. Overall, the data tend to support the conclusion by Akiskal (1990) that dysthymics are more subjectively than objectively depressed yet no less impaired in view of the chronicity of their condition.

Because we tried to exclude secondary dysthymia and also recruited patients from the community, we may have encountered a sample of patients who are more representative of dysthymia in the general population. Overall our data paint the picture of a low-grade lifelong disorder: early onset (perhaps going back to childhood), chronicity with a long and unremitting course, low-grade depression, but, despite this, high levels of impairment. These considerations cohere with those formulated by Akiskal (1983).

Assessment

The levels of impairment were measured with the Sheehan Disabilities Scale at screen (Work: mean = 6.5, SD = 1.5; Social Activities: mean = 7.5, SD = 1.4; Family/Home: mean = 8.8, SD = 2.8). The Social Adjustment Scale mean was 2.8 (SD = 0.7). As Akiskal (1990) states, many of these patients seem to direct all the energy they have toward work. Kraepelin (1921) described this as follows: "Life with its activity is a burden which they habitually bear with dutiful self-denial without being compensated by the pleasure(s) of existence."

The Hamilton Rating Scale for Depression (mean = 20.5, SD = 1.8) was only moderately raised. The question is whether the Hamilton scale is adequate to assess the symptoms and impairments of these patients. This scale is based mainly on vegetative symptoms, classically present in episodic or "endogenous" depression, and it may not be the appropriate means to assess dysthymia.

Outcome

It is generally stated in the literature that the outcome of dysthymic patients is not good, and at least it is much worse than that of major depression (Howland, 1991). The outcome data, recently summarized by Akiskal and Weise (1992), are based largely on double depressives. There are actually few studies addressing the issue of the outcome of adequately treated dysthymia (Kocsis et al., 1991).

Our studies followed up a total of 276 patients with dysthymia for 6 years. The patients were treated with medications to test the therapeutic value of classical and new thymoleptic agents.

The study with moclobemide was a double-blind comparison with imipramine and placebo (Versiani, 1994). Mean dosages (in milligrams) were as follows: moclobemide, 674 (SD = 117); imipramine, 219 (SD = 45); placebo (tablets), 4.8 (SD = 0.5). No formal psychotherapy was associated, nor were other specific psychological interventions. The study was part of a multicenter study of dysthymics from Latin American centers. The results, basically, have shown a significant drug effect (statistical and clinical) in approximately 70% of the patients, compared with 20% in the placebo group. Both medications, moclobemide and imipramine, were similar in efficacy. These results compare favorably with those obtained in trials with major depression.

The 120 patients from the double-blind study were openly followed up with moclobemide to 6 years with good results. Another group of 156 patients were also openly followed up to 6 years either with tranyl-cypromine or with a capsule combining amitriptyline and chlordiazepox-ide. Mean dosages were 44 (SD = 4.6) mg/day for tranylcypromine and 5.2 (SD = 1.3) caps/day for amitriptyline plus chlordiazepoxide (each caps = amitriptyline 12.5 mg + chlordiazepoxide 5 mg). Both medications were effective in two out of three patients.

Long-term treatment studies in dysthymia have been mainly uncontrolled with "naturalistic" methodologies (Howland, 1991). Kocsis et al. (1996) defend a maintenance treatment of at least 2 years, and possibly indefinitely, as do Akiskal et al. (1980). Accordingly, our study of 276 patients was initially maintained on pharmacotherapy for 2 years. Fifty-six patients (21.9%) dropped out. It was decided to withdraw medication after 2 years. This procedure, however, led to a great deal of relapse (89.1%), and the treatment had to be reinstituted for another 2 years; 4-year data will be reported elsewhere; and a fuller report of our study will appear elsewhere.

Conclusion

Our sample consisted of long-standing dysthymics who, even after closer examination, could not say exactly when their disorder started. The majority of our patients initially fulfilled criteria for depressive personality according to Schneider (1959) and as operationalized by Akiskal (1990). With thymoleptic treatment, though, they felt a major difference in their lives. The following is a typical statement by a patient: "I thought I was a sad person, now I feel different, it is as if life is a rich experience I had never felt before."

Such patient testimonials to the efficacy of pharmacotherapy were associated with at least 70% drop in the Hamilton, Social Adjustment, and Disabilities scales. However, the medications were not necessarily miraculous. Many patients dropped out because of unwanted medication effects; moclobemide appeared the least problematic from this standpoint.

Because this was a therapeutic study, we cannot address questions on the validation of dysthymia. Real validation can only come out of "external" validators such as those delineated by Akiskal et al. (1980). Nor do our data permit discussion of dysthymia versus depressive personality. What our data do point out, however, is that these patients (DSM-III-R dysthymics) may profit significantly from antidepressant medication that has been used in systematic trials (old monoamine oxidase inhibitors [MAOIs], new MAOIs, or tricyclics), and the benefits are such that their lives are often entirely transformed.

Although our data cannot resolve questions on the nosological validity of the diagnosis of dysthymia, we can assert that it is important to subsume this construct under mood disorders to bring the therapeutic benefits of thymoleptic agents to a large number of patients who have been traditionally considered pharmacotherapy resistant. Finally, we wish to point out that placebo responses were very low in our sample, which means spontaneous recovery is unlikely in this group of depressions with long-standing "low-level" depression. Overall, our data support the initial findings by Akiskal et al. (1980) on the substantial utility of thymoleptic agents in this special subgroup of chronically depressed individuals.

References

Akiskal, H. S. (1983). Dysthymic disorder: Psychopathology of proposed chronic depressive subtypes. *American Journal of Psychiatry, 140,* 11–20.

Akiskal, H. S. (1990). Toward a definition of dysthymia: Boundaries with personality and mood disorders. In S. W. Burton & H. S. Akiskal (Eds.), *Dysthymic disorder* (pp. 1–12). London: Gaskell.

Akiskal, H. S., Rosenthal, T. L., Haykal, R. F., Lemmi, H., Rosenthal, R. H., & Scott-Strauss, A. (1980). Characterological depressions: Clinical and sleep EEG findings separating "subaffective dysthymias" from "character spectrum disorders." *Archives of General Psychiatry, 37,* 777–783.

Akiskal, H. S., & Weise, R. E. (1992). The clinical spectrum of so-called "minor" depression. *American Journal of Psychotherapy, 46,* 9–22.

American Psychiatric Association. (1987). *Diagnostic and statistical manual of mental disorders* (3rd ed., rev.). Washington, DC: Author.

Derogatis, L. R., Lipman, R. S., & Covi, L. (1973). SCL-90: An outpatient psychiatric rating scale—preliminary report. *Psychopharmacology Bulletin, 9,* 13–28.

Hamilton, M. (1959). The assessment of anxiety scales by rating. *British Journal of Medical Psychology, 32,* 50–55.

Howland, R. H. (1991). Pharmacotherapy of dysthymia: A review. *Journal of Clinical Psychopharmacology, 11,* 83–92.

Keller, M. B., & Shapiro, R. W. (1982). "Double depression": Superimposition of acute depressive episodes on chronic depressive disorders. *American Journal of Psychiatry, 139,* 438–442.

Kocsis, J. H., & Frances, A. J. (1987). A critical discussion of DSM-III dysthymic disorder. *American Journal of Psychiatry, 144,* 1534–1542.

Kocsis, J. H., Frances, A. J., Voss, C., Mann, J. J., Mason, B. J., & Sweeney, J. (1988). Imipramine treatment for chronic depression. *Archives of General Psychiatry, 45,* 253–257.

Kocsis, J. H., Friedman, R. A., Markowitz, J. C., Leon, A. C., Miller, N. L., Gniwesch, L., & Parides, L. (1996) Maintenance therapy for chronic depression: A controlled trial of desipramine. *Archives of General Psychiatry, 53,* 769–774.

Kocsis, J. H., Sutton, B. M., & Frances, A. J. (1991). Long-term follow-up of chronic depression treated with imipramine. *Journal of Clinical Psychiatry, 52,* 56–59.

Kocsis, J. H., Voss, C., Mann, J. J., & Frances, A. (1986). Chronic depression: Demographic and clinical characteristics. *Psychopharmacology Bulletin, 22,* 192–195.

Kraepelin, E. (1921). *Manic–depressive insanity and paranoia* (R. M. Barclay, Trans.; G. M. Robertson, Ed.). Edinburgh: Livingstone.

Schneider, K. (1959). *Clinical psychopathology.* New York: Grune and Stratton.

Sheehan, D. V. (1986). *The anxiety disease.* New York: Charles Scribner's Sons.

Spitzer, R., Williams, J. B., & Gibbon, M. (1987). *Structured Clinical Interview for DSM-III-R (SCID I and II).* New York: New York State Psychiatric Institute.

Versiani, M. (1994). Pharmacotherapy of dysthymia: A controlled study with imipramine, moclobemide or placebo. *Neuropsychopharmacology, 10*(3S1), S-62-266.

Versiani, M., Gentil, V., Guz, J., & et al. (1986). Data about 508 cases of panic disorder and responses to treatment with alprazolam, clomipramine, imipramine and tranylcypromine. In C. Shagass & et al. (Eds.), *Biological psychiatry 1985* (pp. 687–689). Amsterdam: Elsevier.

Versiani, M., Nardi, A. E., Mundim, F. D., Alves, A. B., Liebowitz, M. R., & Amrein, R. (1992). Pharmacotherapy of social phobia: A controlled study with moclobemide and phenelzine. *British Journal of Psychiatry, 161,* 353–360.

Weissman, M. M., Prusoff, B. A., Thompson, W. D., Harding, P. S., & Myers, J. K. (1978). Social adjustment by self-report in a community sample and in psychiatric outpatients. *Journal of Nervous and Mental Disease, 166,* 317–326.

CHAPTER 3

Primary Dysthymia: Predictors of Treatment Response

Arun V. Ravindran
Yvon D. Lapierre

The diagnostic category of dysthymic disorder was introduced in DSM-III (American Psychiatric Association, 1980) to encompass all chronic low-grade depressions, replacing the older concept of neurotic depression, and to include patients who, in the past, were described by several overlapping but not necessarily synonymous terms such as "depressive temperament," "reactive depression," and "chronic minor depression." Subsequently, in DSM-III-R (American Psychiatric Association, 1987), dysthymic disorder was refined to exclude major depression with partial remission and to define primary–secondary and early–late onset subtypes. Primary dysthymia is a low-grade depression lasting more than 2 years. It usually has an insidious onset beginning in childhood or adolescence with a persistent or intermittent course and concurrent "character" pathology. Occasionally, its onset is in early adult life (late onset). Secondary dysthymia develops as a consequence of a chronic disorder of a physical or psychological nature.

The DSM-III-R classification of chronic depressions was influenced to a large extent by the nosological framework developed by Akiskal for this heterogeneous group of patients (Akiskal, 1981, 1983). Scott (1988) proposed a similar classification and suggested the addition of "double depression," which is the superimposition of an acute depressive episode on dysthymia as another group (Keller & Shapiro, 1982). DSM-IV (American Psychiatric Association, 1994) has essentially endorsed these ideas, with one important exception: The primary–secondary distinction has been deleted. This is unfortunate, because, as we hope to demonstrate in this chapter, primary dysthymia—and its subtypes—may embody important treatment implications.

The Classification of Dysthymic Disorders

Akiskal et al. (1981) reported that primary dysthymia constituted about one-third (37%) of all depressions in a community mental health center. These patients showed many symptoms of depression, including anhedonia, sleep disturbance, poor self-esteem, guilty ruminations, hopelessness, and suicidal ideation, as well as fatigue and other psychomotor symptoms. The symptoms usually fluctuated in intensity, remaining less severe than in major depression but with a more persistent or an intermittent course. Because patients with dysthymia show character difficulties, they often have been considered to have a characterological depression and traditionally have been treated with psychotherapy.

More recently, Akiskal (1983, 1990) proposed that primary dysthymia be further subdivided into two distinct subgroups, character spectrum disorder (CSD) and subaffective dysthymia (SD). The SD subtype is seen as a mild chronic primary mood disorder. It has presenting symptoms characteristic of major depression—at a subsyndromal level—frequently with a family history of depression, and it usually responds well to antidepressant therapy. It is thought to have a predisposing constitutional or biological depressive substrate. The CSD subtype includes patients with depressive symptoms and significant personality pathology, polydrug and alcohol abuse, and familial alcoholism, and this subgroup shows a poor response to pharmacotherapy.

Akiskal's framework is supported by Rihmer (1990), although others (Murphy & Checkley, 1990) have questioned its validity (Murphy, 1991). The latter authors found no significant differences between the two subtypes of primary dysthymia in treatment response to a serotonergic agent, noting significant improvement in both groups.

Although there may be disagreement on the classification of dysthymia, there is a consensus that this illness has significant morbidity. The point prevalence for this disorder is estimated between 3% and 5% of the adult population (Weissman et al., 1988; Goldberg & Bridges, 1990). Dysthymia is associated with increased vulnerability for major depression (Lewinsohn et al., 1991; Markowitz et al., 1992). It is also associated with high utilization of psychiatric and general health care services and increased social morbidity (Weissman et al., 1988; Johnson et al., 1992;

Klerman & Weissman, 1992). However, currently there are no guidelines to assist clinicians in treating this condition.

The goals of our investigation were to further characterize the features of primary dysthymia, to evaluate the effectiveness of selective serotonin reuptake inhibitors (SSRIs) in its treatment, and to attempt to define the predictors of response to treatment.

Predicting Treatment Response

Description of Study

The findings are based on 69 patients who were either physician- or self-referred for evaluation and treatment. Of these 69 patients, 60 completed at least 6 weeks of treatment and 9 dropped out. All had signed an informed consent to participate in the study. They ranged from 18 to 60 years old. Fuller details of this study are given elsewhere (Ravindran et al., 1994).

The diagnostic criteria were those of dysthymia (DSM-III-R) plus Akiskal's criteria for primary dysthymia of the SD versus CSD subtypes. In order to maintain as much homogeneity of the sample as possible, any other Axis I disorder, substance abuse, physical disorder, or interfering physiological condition, such as pregnancy, excluded the patient from the study sample.

The data that were collected included patient characteristics (age, sex, marital status), duration of current episode, presenting and posttreatment symptoms (standardized clinician- and self-rated depression and anxiety scales), and an uncorroborated screening report of family history of Axis I psychiatric illness(es). Clinical ratings were done by three trained psychiatrists who had demonstrated interrater reliability for the assessment instruments used. These were the 17-item Hamilton Rating Scales for Depression (HAM-D; Hamilton, 1967) and Anxiety (HAM-A; Hamilton, 1959) and Clinical Global Evaluation of Improvement (CGI) on a 7-point scale. In addition, a 56-item self-rating instrument, the Hopkins Symptom Checklist (HSCL; Derogatis et al., 1974), was completed by the majority of patients.

Assessments were completed at admission, after a 1-week placebo washout (baseline), and again at least at 1, 2, 4, and 6 weeks of treatment. The baseline and week 6 data were analyzed to determine response to treatment. The criterion for a positive treatment response was a reduction of 50% on the HAM-D, resulting in a final score of 7 or less. In addition, the patient should no longer meet the symptom criteria for dysthymia.

The main groups that were compared were the subgroups of dysthymia (CSD, early onset SD, late onset SD) and patient response to treatment (responders, nonresponders). These groups were compared on the following variables using univariate (t tests, chi-square) analyses; HAM-D and HAM-A (item, factor, and total scores), revised HAM-D and HAM-A[1] scores, HSCL (factor and total scores), CGI, demographic variables, personality traits, and family history of psychiatric illnesses.

Comparison of Subgroups of Primary Dysthymics

Several differences between the subgroups of primary dysthymic patients were noted, and these are shown in Table 3.1. As expected, CSD and early onset SD patients had significantly lower ages of illness onset than did late onset SD patients. The late onset SD patients also tended to be older at the time of treatment. With respect to symptoms, CSD patients self-reported significantly more psychic anxiety than both groups of SD patients. These patients also tended to have higher baseline HAM-D scores than did the late onset SD patients, whereas HAM-D scores for the early onset SD group were in between the other two groups.

Treatment Response

The overall response rate for all primary dysthymic patients was 65%. Significant improvement was noted in both depression and anxiety symptoms, with changes in both types of symptom being highly correlated ($r =$

TABLE 3.1. Comparison of the Subgroups of Primary Dysthymics on Demographic and Baseline Clinical Variables

Variable	CSD ($n = 6$) a	Early onset SD ($n = 46$) b	Late onset SD ($n = 8$) c	Statistical significance[a]
Current age[b]	34.0 ± 13.5	39.8 ± 9.0	46.1 ± 9.2	a < c, $p = .07$
Age at illness onset	16.2 ± 9.1	17.4 ± 6.8	28.0 ± 8.7	ab < c, $p < .01$
% married	60%	39%	43%	ns
Baseline ratings				
HAM-D	19.7 ± 4.2	18.1 ± 3.9	16.0 ± 2.8	a > c, $p = .09$
HAM-A	10.0 ± 2.4	12.2 ± 4.2	9.4 ± 3.7	ns
HSCL factor 5 (Psychic Anxiety)	2.8 ± 0.8	2.0 ± 0.6	1.9 ± 0.8	a > bc, $p < .02$
CGI	3.5 ± 0.5	3.6 ± 0.5	3.5 ± 0.5	ns

[a]Analyses performed with t tests or chi-square test.
[b]Mean $\pm$ SD.

.81; $p < .001$). Similar results were found even when the revised scoring for the HAM-D and HAM-A (Riskind et al., 1987) was used in order to measure pure depression and pure anxiety symptoms independently (i.e., correlation between the change scores was .55; $p < .001$).

The response rates for subgroups of dysthymic patients differed markedly. SD patients had a significantly higher response rate (70.4%) than did CSD patients (16.7%) ($\chi^2[1] = 6.85$, $p < .01$), and most of the dropouts were CSD patients (7/9). As well, a significantly higher percentage of early (76.1%) compared to late (37.5%) onset SD patients responded to antidepressant treatment ($\chi^2[1] = 4.87$, $p < .03$).

Responders had significantly lower mean baseline total scores on the HAM-D ($p = .05$) but not the HAM-A. When depression and anxiety symptoms were measured independently using the revised HAM-D and HAM-A, responders still had significantly lower baseline scores on the HAM-D ($p = .01$) but not the HAM-A.

Higher observer-rated general somatic symptoms (HAM-D item 13; $p = .04$) and self-reported psychic anxiety (HSCL factor 5; $p = .03$) were associated with a poor treatment response. In addition, self-reported psychic anxiety was significantly higher in the CSD patients, who showed a poor response to treatment.

Of the Schneiderian personality traits (see Akiskal, 1983), being gloomy and pessimistic ($p = .06$) or self-critical and self-reproaching ($p = .09$) pointed toward poorer outcome in all patients but reached statistical significance only for the SD group ($p < .05$ for both). Surprisingly, such traits as being skeptical, hypercritical, and complaining or preoccupied with inadequacy and failure did not predict a poor outcome.

There was no difference in current age or gender between responders and nonresponders. However, when the interaction between age and sex was analyzed, the response rate was much higher for male patients older than 40 (73%) than for those 40 or under (44%), although this effect was not significant.

Overall, patients who were married or living common law had a higher response rate (82%) than did patients who were single, separated, divorced, or widowed (58%); however, this effect only reached statistical significance ($p = .04$) for SD patients.

The percentage of patients reporting a family history of depression was quite high, 73%; for alcoholism it was 37%. Responders had a higher incidence of depression in first-degree relatives (77%) than did nonresponders (65%), but this effect did not reach significance. Nonresponders had a higher incidence of alcoholism in their family—mothers (25% vs. 5%; $p = .02$), fathers (50% vs. 26%; $p = .06$), siblings (30% vs. 10%; $p = .05$).

Discussion

Our data support the current classification of primary dysthymia proposed by Akiskal. We found that the response rate was higher in SD than in CSD, although the number of patients in the latter group was small. However, seven of nine dropouts from the study (considered treatment failures by clinical judgment) were also CSD patients. These findings support the view that dysthymic patients with marked character pathology—especially of the dramatic cluster—represent a special challenge to clinicians.[2]

We found the response to be significantly better in early onset compared to late onset SD patients. In major depression, an early age of onset has been associated with both poor long-term prognosis and an increased family history of depressive disorders (Weissman et al., 1984; Price et al., 1987). It may be that the genetic vulnerability differs in the two subgroups of dysthymia, with a greater familial loading indicating a more biological illness and a better response to pharmacotherapy in the early onset patients. However, the reason for the better response in early onset SD patients remains speculative at this time.

In major depression, histrionic, antisocial, and dependent personality traits and the lack of guilt and extrapunitiveness are thought to indicate poor outcome (Bielski & Friedel, 1976; Charney et al., 1981; Pfohl et al., 1984). These traits were common in the CSD group, which showed a poor response to treatment. However, the relationship between personality factors and treatment response in dysthymia may not be as straightforward because the presence of certain traits, such as being skeptical, hypercritical, and complaining or being preoccupied with inadequacy, was not associated with poor outcome in these patients. This finding supports the view that many of these personality characteristics may be related to the chronicity of the illness.

Severity has been associated with good response in major depression, which does not appear to be the case in primary dysthymia, where patients with less severe depression showed a better response to treatment. Over half our sample had HAM-D scores of 17 or greater. One possibility was that the patients with HAM-D scores above 17 were suffering from double depression, although we believe that this is unlikely because none of the patients met the DSM-III-R criteria for major depression. Measurement error may be partly responsible because this scale was developed and validated for use in clinical depression, where symptoms are more sustained and acutely impairing, whereas in dysthymia they tend to vary in intensity, duration, and frequency. Also, the HAM-D is known to be weighted heavily toward anxiety symptoms, and this may have contributed to some of the relatively high severity scores in our sample. It is recognized that in dysthymia, there is variability in the severity of depressive symptoms within the disorder itself. However, there appears to be a need for a specific instrument for dysthymia that is sensitive to the mild fluctuating symptoms of this illness.

We found somatic and psychic anxiety to predict poor outcome. The presence of high anxiety in depression has also been reported to be associated with a poorer response to some antidepressants (Overall et al., 1966; Paykel, 1971).

Our family history data were obtained only by self-report. One important finding was that 73% of patients reported depressive illness among their first-degree relatives, with responders showing a slightly greater family history. Also noteworthy, a greater family history of alcoholism was associated with a poor response to treatment for the whole sample and when SD patients were analyzed separately. These data extend previous findings by Akiskal et al. (1981), who reported that a poor response to antidepressants was associated with a family history of alcoholism, but most of the patients with such family history were CSD.

Clinical Observations

From our experience with primary dysthymic patients, we made the following observations:

- A significant number of primary early onset dysthymics did not show obvious character pathology (such as histrionic, antisocial, and dependent personality traits or drug abuse), characteristics believed to be part of DSM-III dysthymia. Many had achieved a college education or professional degree and functioned reasonably well, despite struggling with fluctuating symptoms. They appear to have developed coping strategies to deal with their day-to-day stressors, often becoming socially withdrawn, overdedicated to work, rigid, and defensive in attitude.
- A common complaint from these patients was that they had lacked "the spark of life" since their early teens, and they had to work very hard to achieve what they have accomplished in life. The treatment response was dramatic for many (often occurring within 3 to 4 weeks), with patients expressing that they were experiencing a sense of well-being for the first time in their life. They were concerned that this novel emotion of euthymia may be transient until they were reassured.
- Most patients who attempted to withdraw from medication opted to go back on it when their symptoms returned. Preliminary exami-

nation of our 2-year follow-up records suggests that many primary early onset dysthymic patients may need long-term, or possibly lifetime, maintenance medication.

Conclusion

Dysthymia is a mood disorder with significant morbidity, and recent research indicates that many patients with dysthymia may benefit from pharmacotherapy. Akiskal's proposed subtyping of primary dysthymia comes closest to offering guidelines for antidepressant prediction in this illness. However, there is an obvious need for further research on the biological substrate(s) of this disorder to develop more objective measures for predicting the optimal treatment modality for an individual patient.

Acknowledgments

The authors wish to thank R. J. Bialik, PhD, for help with data analyses, and C. Waddell, RN, for coordination and management of the patients during the treatment phases.

Notes

1. The scores from the HAM-D and HAM-A were rescored using the method of Riskind et al. (1987) to produce revised scores thought to measure pure anxiety and depression symptoms. Our data indicated that although the HAM-D and HAM-A were highly correlated with each other ($r = .64$; $p < .001$), the revised scales were not significantly correlated ($r = .06$; $p = .34$), indicating that the scales were measuring different symptoms.

2. Editors' note: That "character spectrum" patients do not respond well to antidepressants does not, of course, imply that they are beyond all pharmacotherapy. Anticycling agents appear relevant to these patients (see Akiskal, Chapter 1, this volume).

References

Akiskal, H. S. (1981). Subaffective disorders: Dysthymic, cyclothymic and bipolar II disorders in the "borderline" realm. *Psychiatric Clinics of North America, 4,* 25–46.

Akiskal, H. S. (1983). Dysthymic disorder: Psychopathology of proposed chronic depressive subtypes. *American Journal of Psychiatry, 140*(1), 11–20.

Akiskal, H. S. (1990). Towards a definition of dysthymia: Boundaries with personality and mood disorders. In S. W. Burton & H. S. Akiskal (Eds.), *Dysthymic disorder* (pp. 1–12). London: Gaskell.

Akiskal, H. S., King, D., Rosenthal, T. L., Robinson, D., & Scott-Strauss, A. (1981). Chronic depressions. Part 1. Clinical and familial characteristics in 137 probands. *Journal of Affective Disorders, 3,* 297–315.

American Psychiatric Association. (1980). *Diagnostic and statistical manual of mental disorders* (3rd ed.). Washington, DC: Author.

American Psychiatric Association. (1987). *Diagnostic and statistical manual of mental disorders* (3rd ed., rev.). Washington, DC: Author.

Bielski, R. J., & Friedel, R. O. (1976). Prediction of tricyclic antidepressant response: A critical review. *Archives of General Psychiatry, 33,* 1479–1489.

Charney, D. S., Nelson, J. C., & Quinlan, D. M. (1981). Personality traits and disorder in depression. *American Journal of Psychiatry, 138,* 1601–1604.

Derogatis, L. R., Lipman, R. S., Rickels, K., Uhlenhuth, E. H., & Covi, L. (1974). The Hopkins Symptoms Checklist (HSCL): A measure of primary symptom dimensions. *Modern Problems of Pharmacopsychiatry, 7,* 79–110.

Goldberg, D. P., & Bridges, K. W. (1990). Epidemiological observations on the concept of dysthymic disorder. In S. W. Burton & H. S. Akiskal (Eds.), *Dysthymic disorder* (pp. 104–111). London: Gaskell.

Hamilton, M. (1959). The assessment of anxiety states by rating. *British Journal of Medical Psychology, 32,* 50–55.

Hamilton, M. (1967). Development of a rating scale for primary depressive illness. *British Journal of Social and Clinical Psychology, 6,* 278–296.

Johnson, J., Weissman, M. M., & Klerman, G. L. (1992). Service utilization and social morbidity associated with depressive symptoms in the community. *Journal of the American Medical Association, 267,* 1478–1483.

Keller, M. B., & Shapiro, R. W. (1982). "Double depression": Superimposition of acute depressive episodes on chronic depressive disorders. *American Journal of Psychiatry, 139,* 438–442.

Klerman, G. L., & Weissman, M. M. (1992). The course, morbidity, and costs of depression. *Archives of General Psychiatry, 49,* 831–834.

Lewinsohn, P. M., Rohde, P., Seeley, J. R., & Hops, H. (1991). Comorbidity of unipolar depression: I. Major depression with dysthymia. *Journal of Abnormal Psychology, 100,* 205–213.

Markowitz, J. C., Moran, M. E., Kocsis, J. H., & Frances, A. J. (1992). Prevalence and comorbidity of dysthymic disorder among psychiatric outpatients. *Journal of Affective Disorders, 24,* 63–71.

Murphy, D. G. M. (1991). The classification and treatment of dysthymia. *British Journal of Psychiatry, 158,* 106–109.

Murphy, D., & Checkley, S. A. (1990). Dysthymia presenting to the Emergency Clinic at the Maudsley Hospital. In S. W. Burton & H. S. Akiskal (Eds.), *Dysthymic disorder* (pp. 37–48). London: Gaskell.

Overall, J. E., Hollister, L. E., Johnson, M., & Pennington, V. (1966). Nosology of depression and differential response to drugs. *Journal of the American Medical Association, 195,* 946–948.

Paykel, E. S. (1971). Classification of depressed patients: A cluster analysis derived grouping. *British Journal of Psychiatry, 118,* 275–288.

Pfohl, B., Stangl, D., & Zimmerman, M. (1984). The implications of DSM-III personality disorders for patients with major depression. *Journal of Affective Disorders, 7,* 309–318.

Price, R. A., Kidd, K. K., & Weissman, M. M. (1987). Early onset (under age 30 years) and panic disorder as markers for etiologic homogeneity in major depression. *Archives of General Psychiatry, 44,* 434–440.

Ravindran, A. V., Bialik, R. J., & Lapierre, Y. D. (1994). Therapeutic efficacy of specific serotonin reuptake inhibitors (SSRIs) in dysthymia. *Canadian Journal of Psychiatry, 39,* 21-26.

Rihmer, Z. (1990). Dysthymia: A clinician's perspective. In S.W. Burton & H.S. Akiskal (Eds.), *Dysthymic disorder* (pp. 112–125). London: Gaskell.

Riskind, J. H., Beck, A. T., Brown, G., & Steer, R. A. (1987). Taking the measure of anxiety and depression: Validity of the reconstructed Hamilton scales. *Journal of Nervous and Mental Disease, 175,* 474–479.

Scott, J. (1988). Chronic depression. *British Journal of Psychiatry, 153,* 287–297.

Weissman, M. M., Leaf, P. J., Bruce, M. L., & Florio, L. (1988). The epidemiology of dysthymia in five communities: Rates, risks, comorbidity, and treatment. *American Journal of Psychiatry, 145,* 815–819.

Weissman, M. M., Wickramaratne, P., Merikangas, K. R., Leckman, J. F., Prusoff, B. A., Caruso, K. A., Kidd, K. K., & Gammon, G. D. (1984). Onset of major depression in early adulthood. Increased familial loading and specificity. *Archives of General Psychiatry, 41,* 1136–1143.

CHAPTER 4

Chronic and Residual Major Depressions

Giovanni B. Cassano
Mario Savino

Spontaneously remitting symptomatology with periodic course during which episodes of illness alternate with symptom-free intervals was traditionally considered a major characteristic of mood disorders, carrying important diagnostic implications as far as its differentiation from characteristics of schizophrenic and personality disorders were concerned. However, since Kraepelin's (1913) early observations, reports have been published of chronic, unremitting depressive conditions (Akiskal et al., 1981; Scott et al., 1988), and, more recently, the adoption of the concept of a broader spectrum of mood disorders has indicated that chronicity might involve the entire realm, from unipolar (Akiskal et al., 1981) to bipolar (Akiskal, 1996) illness and from subclinical to full-blown melancholia. Even though the bipolar spectrum disorders in our collaborative Pisa–Memphis studies (Akiskal et al., 1989) were grouped in episodic and persistent forms, a wide range of mild subclinical long-lasting manifestations covers the interval as a bridge between the two classes of affective disorders. Table 4.1 lists the chronic forms within this spectrum.

Continuity and Chronicity of Depression

Continuity and chronicity represent important features of mood disorders, which appear as enduring illnesses, often subgrouped on the basis of periodic severe exacerbations yet springing out as full-blown episodes from

TABLE 4.1. The Spectrum of Chronicity in Depression

Depressive temperament
Dysthymia
Residual depressive symptoms
Chronic major depressive episode
Brief recurrent depression
Protracted mixed depression
Predominantly depressive rapid cycling
Chronic maladjustment with depressive mood
Chronic comorbid conditions with depressive mood
Chronic depression secondary to physical disorders

an affective temperamental background, followed by long-standing residual symptoms. Clinical observation, accurate anamnestic records, and prolonged follow-up demonstrate how temperament, major and minor depressions, protracted mixed states, high-frequency recurrences, residual symptoms, and chronic maladjustment determine continuous or partially intermittent conditions in which depressive manifestations prevail.

Thus, short- or long-lasting major syndromes usually overlap with minor isolated signs and symptoms, as well as maladaptive—and sometimes, superadaptive—traits, which testify to the continuity of an underlying psychopathological process involving, respectively, depressive and hyperthymic temperamental terrains. This consideration has relevant clinical implications for both diagnosis and treatment. The remission of a major episode can be due to appropriate treatment as well as to spontaneous course of the illness, so that the major task for the clinician is accurate diagnosis and follow-up of the patient. The reported efficacy of nonspecific agents such as benzodiazepines—and psychotherapy—has to be examined in a long-term perspective. Moreover, patient compliance with medication, especially in bipolar patients, has to be ensured for the euthymic phase to be reached. Psychosocial stressors have to be evaluated against the background of a constitution that predisposes the patient to marked reactions to a large spectrum of possible "depressant" factors, and, often, the peculiar temperamental characteristics are in themselves capable of enhancing the frequency and severity of stressors.

Mood disorders as chronic illnesses have to be carefully assessed in order to obtain a comprehensive view for the clinician who meets the patient during the full-blown index episode. The entire mood spectrum, from familial data and temperament to major syndromic features, plus lifetime and intraepisodic comorbid conditions, will constitute a detailed picture of the patient whom the clinician is expected to treat and follow up.

Comorbidity and Chronicity

Since Feinstein's (1970) observations on co-occurring chronic physical diseases, chronicity and comorbidity have shown close links. The presence of comorbidity phenomena carries a great risk of protraction of the course of depression (VanValkenburg et al., 1984; Coryell et al., 1988), and such long-standing mood disorders as dysthymia show very high rates of comorbidity (Weissman et al., 1988). "Neurotic," "characterological," and "atypical" depressions were considered chronic subtypes of mood disorders or lifelong personality disorders until the comorbidity approach and the concept of mood and anxiety spectra forced clinical researchers to nosographical reassessment, with important diagnostic and therapeutic implications.

The impact of comorbidity on the features of depression is summarized in Table 4.2. The presence of comorbid disorders, even as mild spectrum manifestations, can account for several forms of "atypical" presentation of depressive conditions. This diagnostic approach to long-standing conditions allows clinicians to better evaluate the reciprocal influences of co-occurring disorders either in their full-blown or their minor–atypical symptomatological expressions, and thus can help in optimizing treatment choices.

Chronicity in Clinical Populations

Each depressive condition can show a protracted course, and severity of depression can fluctuate in the same patient. Figure 4.1 diagrams a prototypical life-chart course of "chronic depressive illness" by the representation of its various components.

TABLE 4.2. Clinical Subtypes of Depression as a Function of Comorbidity

Clinical presentation	Comorbid disorders
Anxious depression	Generalized anxiety disorder Panic–agoraphobic spectrum
Neurasthenia	Panic–agoraphobic spectrum Somatoform disorders Obsessive–compulsive spectrum Infectious and other physical disorders
Atypical depression	Panic–agoraphobic spectrum Somatoform disorders Eating disorders Social phobia Obsessive–compulsive spectrum

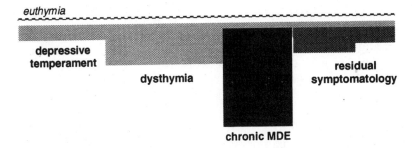

FIGURE 4.1. Diagrammatic representation of the spectrum of protracted depressive conditions.

If we keep together the rates of the mild protracted depressive conditions in our study population (Cassano et al., 1989), full-blown depression rarely appears as a well-delimited entity on a euthymic background, even in clinical populations selected by restrictive exclusion criteria. Table 4.3 reports the percentages of long-standing depressive conditions and temperamental dysregulations in a large sample of major depressives; despite the exclusion of physical diseases and comorbid mental disorders, patients selected by the presence of a clear-cut DSM-III-R "primary" major depressive episode (MDE; American Psychiatric Association, 1987) often have suffered from several other manifestations of the depressive spectrum. Comparing different subtypes of MDE, chronicity appears pertinent to the entire mood disorder spectrum, unipolar as well as bipolar subtypes.

Chronicity in Major Depressive Subtypes

Despite its characteristic tendency to spontaneous remission, MDE can assume a very protracted course. Chronic depressions are reported in

TABLE 4.3. Protracted Depressive Conditions among 527 patients with Different Subtypes of Mood Disorder Presenting with Index MDE (DSM-III-R)

MDE subtypes	Depressive temperament (%)	Chronic MDE (%)	Residual symptoms (%)
Unipolar (n = 408)	41.2	19.5	45.8
Bipolar II (n = 90)	19.1	13.3	37.9
Bipolar I (n = 29)	40.0	11.4	24.9
Total for entire sample	38.0	18.2	36.1

4–28% of cases (Robins & Guze, 1972); lower rates are recorded in short-term follow-up and during pharmacological trials requiring such strict admission criteria as circumscribed age span, exclusion of physical and mental comorbid conditions, and absence of previous treatments.

In our study (Musetti et al., 1987), chronicity is most frequent among single major episode depressives. Although all diagnostic MDE subtypes can have a chronic denouement, spontaneous switches and greater tendency to cycling with frequent recurrences might account for the lower chronicity rates recorded among bipolar depressives.

So-called poorer prognosis, the atypical symptomatology, and frequent resistance to treatment have, in the past, delineated these long-standing MDEs as distinct subtypes among mood disorders, with ill-defined boundaries toward schizophrenic and personality disorders. The reported stability of the rates of chronic MDE during the past three decades, despite the availability of new effective antidepressant treatments, continues to be a formidable challenge to the clinician.

Chronic versus Nonchronic Major Depressive Episodes

Findings from several studies (Akiskal, 1982; Musetti et al., 1987) show that chronic and nonchronic MDE share most symptomatological, biological, and familial characteristics. Thus, chronic depressions have rapid eye movement latency and response to the desamethazone suppression test similar to those of nonchronic depression, supporting the view of chronic MDE as a possible evolution of the MDE rather than a different diagnostic entity, carrying greater therapeutic problems and requiring a more complex and well-designed management. Our sample of 527 depressives did not show substantial differences if compared by different length of the index MDE (Savino et al., 1989) as far as most demographic and diagnostic characteristics (Table 4.4).

The foregoing considerations suggest that clinicians treating chronic MDE must engage in a thorough and systematic evaluation. The first step will be the identification of those depressive syndromes originating and/or maintained by such iatrogenic factors as sedative drugs and neuroleptics, as well as corticosteroids and antihypertensives, and by inappropriate drug combinations. In the recent literature (Scott, 1988), the main predictors of chronicity in MDE are reported to be female sex, old age, unipolar course of the illness, loaded family history, concurrent stressors and premorbid temperamental characteristics, and comorbidity with psychiatric and physical illnesses as originally reported by Akiskal (1982). Another predictor of chronic course is the length of past episodes: Thus, chronic or protracted

TABLE 4.4. Comparison of MDE by Duration of Index Episodes

	>24 months (n = 95)	6–24 months (n = 199)	6 months (n = 233)	p
Males (%)	33.7	34.2	27.9	ns
Mean age (years)	53.3	51.7	48.9	< .05
Stressors (%)	68.4	56.6	48.5	< .05
Mean age at onset (years)	41.1	40.5	39.7	ns
Number of depressive episodes	3.1	3.7	4.9	ns
Number of manic episodes	0.2	0.1	0.2	ns
Mean total HAM-D score	21.4	20.8	21.6	ns

MDE is related to the risk of chronicity of recurrencies (Kerr et al., 1972; Nystrom, 1979; Hirschfeld et al., 1986).

Temperament and Chronicity

The relationships between premorbid temperamental affective dysregulations and chronicity have been a long-standing focus of interest, and the inclusion of these temperamental pathologies among the spectrum of mood disorders is attracting a growing interest because of their relevant diagnostic and prognostic implications.

Premorbid characteristics have often been considered related to the tendency to unremitting course in depressive illness. Thus, neuroticism, histrionic traits (Kerr et al., 1972; Nystrom, 1979), and depressive temperament (Akiskal et al., 1981) have been reported as premorbid characteristics of chronic depressives. A patient's history characterized by such traits could be due to comorbid spectrum phenomena from anxiety, obsessive eating, or somatoform disorders. In our studies, we utilized Akiskal and Mallya's (1987) criteria to assess premorbid temperament; information from both patient and relatives is combined in order to minimize bias. Our data (Cassano et al., 1992) suggest that the hyperthymic temperament might protect against chronicity, being more common among short MDEs; depressive temperament is more frequent among chronic major depressives when compared to nonchronic patients, albeit nonsignificantly, and is related to early onset and high rate of recurrence of superimposed MDE. The relationships between the depressive temperament and dysthymia, double depression, and brief recurrent depression represent fruitful research efforts to paint a more comprehensive picture of the wide mood disorder spectrum (see Klein & Miller, Chapter 7, this volume).

Stressors and Chronicity

Stressors preceding the onset of long-standing depressions have been frequently reported in the literature: Both Akiskal (1982) and Scott et al. (1988) recorded rates of 40–60% of relevant life events of loss before and after the onset of a chronic MDE. The presence of stressors as triggering and maintaining factors of chronic depression appears to be significantly higher in chronic MDE than in MDE shorter than 2 years. In our recent analyses, the percentage of patients reporting stressors before the index episode significantly increased with the length of the episode, reaching a rate of 67.2% among patients with chronic depression (Table 4.5). Even the comparison between chronic and nonchronic MDE, given the limit of 2 or more years of episode's duration (Table 4.4), clearly shows the statistically significant higher frequency of stressors among chronic major depressives.

Chronic MDE and Residual Symptomatology

The growing consensus on the concept of residual symptomatology is widening the area of chronicity among mood disorders and prompting a less strict conceptualization of their periodicity, cyclicity, and tendency to spontaneous full recovery. The clinical observation of residual symptomatology following full-blown episodes, with severe long-lasting maladjustment, further enlarges the concept of chronicity and continuity in mood disorders and highlights the importance of effective long-term treatment of these conditions. These considerations have a great impact on the therapeutic approach to the "major" mood disorders; the detection of residual symptoms and the tendency toward recurrences appear to be influential in long-term maintenance treatment.

In Table 4.5, the rates of residual symptoms following past episodes in our sample reveal a trend to increase with the duration of the index episode. This finding could suggest relationships between residual symptoms and chronic course in MDE. Frequently, long-lasting depression is

TABLE 4.5. Stressors and Residual Symptoms by Different Length of Index MDE in 527 Major Depressives

	1–3 months (n = 153)	3–6 months (n = 80)	6–24 months (n = 199)	> 24 months (n = 95)	p
Stressors (%)	51.4	46.3	55.9	67.2	< .01
Residual symptoms (%)	27.6	40.5	43.0	44.7	< .01

followed by a persistent mild symptomatology characterized by cognitive impairment, mood instability, emotional dyscontrol, and hypersensitivity to negative events with social and work impairment. Residual symptoms often worsen the prognosis, and the treatment should be directed also to these "lesser" manifestations of depressive illness in order to obtain a complete remission and an effective prevention of recurrences.

Clinical Presentation

Several major nuclear symptoms of depression, such as diurnal variation, early awakening, psychomotor retardation, loss of interest, and anhedonia, tend to attenuate when depression takes a long-lasting course; the resulting atypical phenomenology increases the risk of inappropriate diagnoses. Actually, anxiety symptoms often tend to dominate the self-evaluated profile of chronic depression, whereas melancholic features tend to vanish (Cassano et al., 1983). The index cross-sectional evaluation of the clinical picture might lead the practitioner to overlook endogenous features of the disorder, favoring wrong diagnoses. In particular, the mild affective symptomatology of chronic low-grade depressive conditions has led to diagnostic and therapeutic errors. Thus, chronic depressions have also been considered a complication of a preexisting character disorder, or a reaction to acute stressors or to permanently disabling existential conditions.

The accumulating data in the field indicate that enhanced "mood reactivity" to life events, high "rejection sensitivity," a low threshold of frustration to slight stressors, and enduring mild downregulation of mood despite its low symptomatic severity are, nonetheless, to be considered clinical and subclinical expressions of an endogenous process (see, for further elaboration, Akiskal, Chapter 1, and Stewart & Klein, Chapter 12, this volume).

In a previous study on 176 patients with MDE as the index episode (Musetti et al., 1987), we found that 22 (12.5%) had a chronic course (> 2 years). This subgroup shared most features with those patients who had a shorter length of illness. However, chronic major depressives showed higher rates of stressors preceding the index episode, less frequent incongruent psychotic symptoms, and higher scores of the factor "depression" at the self-reported Hopkins Symptom Checklist-90 (Derogatis et al., 1973). This latter characteristic supports Scott et al.'s (1988) observation of worse Beck Depression Inventory scores in patients with long-lasting MDE. Our more recent data on chronic MDE (Table 4.4), once again, shares most features with the acute illness, which means that the clinician has to treat chronic depression vigorously with appropriate somatic treatments.

Comparing clinical samples of dysthymics and chronic major depressives (Table 4.6), major differences were linked to dysthymia's early onset and to definitional differences in depressive symptoms by the Hamilton Rating Scale for Depression (HAM-D; Hamilton, 1967) (Cassano & Savino, 1993). However, dysthymia does represent a disabling condition in terms of duration of illness, social and work impairment (Perugi et al., 1988), and risk for substance abuse and suicide attempts (Akiskal et al., 1981).

Thus, despite their milder severity in cross-sectional clinical presentation, minor chronic depressions produce impairment and risk of severe complications. As summarized in other chapters (see, for instance, Akiskal, Chapter 1, and Ravindran & Lapierre, Chapter 3, this volume), they deserve and benefit from competent psychopharmacotherapy.

Conclusion

Data from systematic studies and observation from clinical practice are painting a picture of mood disorders as enduring illnesses in which chronicity does not necessarily mean persistence of symptomatology on a daily basis. This kind of approach has been strengthened and widened by the usefulness of the concept of a mood disorder spectrum embracing the full range of mood dysregulation, from mild temperamental pathology to major depressive illness and mixed/manic episodes. Chronic full-blown episodes can evolve from any diagnostic subtype of mood disorder, sharing typical symptomatological characteristics with acute major depressive illness.

Dysthymia and prolonged minor mood disorders—as well as chronic major depression—obviously carry greater diagnostic and therapeutic challenges than does acute depression. The vanishing of melancholic features after years of illness, the frequent comorbidity phenomena, and the presence of iatrogenic complications such as benzodiazepine dependence can complicate the clinical presentation of these depressions, which

TABLE 4.6. Dysthymia versus Chronic Major Depression

	Dysthymia ($n = 45$)	Unipolar chronic major depression ($n = 99$)	p
Mean age (years)	42.5	52.9	< .05
Mean age at onset (years)	32.1	41.3	< .05
Males (%)	33.3	30.3	ns
Early onset (< 21 years) (%)	34.1	4.0	< .05
Depressive temperament (%)	28.9	38.4	ns
Suicide attempts (%)	4.4	12.1	ns
HAM-D score	15.7	21.8	< .05

might be considered long-standing episodic manifestations of a chronic illness even in the absence of unremitting underlying temperamental dysregulations and/or residual symptoms. Thus, an accurate diagnostic procedure that takes into account the spectrum and comorbidity concepts on an intraepisodic and lifetime basis will be the prerequisite for the correct management of these conditions.

Therapeutic strategies should, therefore, consider even attenuated low-grade affective conditions as belonging to the mood disorders spectrum; effective doses of antidepressants should be prescribed for long-term treatment, and electroconvulsive therapy used when needed. Bipolar signs will be considered relevant to therapeutic choices, and the tendency of benzodiazepines and neuroleptics to induce chronicization of depression will be minimized by shortening the duration of their utilization (Akiskal & Mallya, 1987). Comorbid conditions are best controlled by "transnosological" thymoleptics—such as the selective serotonin reuptake inhibitors—which can be effective for both disorders; alternatively, well-targeted pharmacological combinations should be used creatively. In that way, compliance with a long-lasting full-dose treatment will be strengthened, even in maintenance therapy during relatively quiescent phases. Such approaches to chronic depression, by optimizing the utilization of old and newer effective antidepressant and mood-stabilizing agents, will further increase clinicians' chances to successfully manage those chronic depressive conditions whose prognosis has traditionally been considered poor.

References

Akiskal, H. S. (1982). Factors associated with incomplete recovery in primary depressive illness. *Journal of Clinical Psychiatry, 43,* 266–271.

Akiskal, H. S. (1996). The prevalent clinical spectrum of bipolar disorders: Beyond DSM-IV. *Journal of Clinical Psychopharmacology, 6*(Suppl. 1), 4S–14S.

Akiskal, H. S., Cassano, G. B., Musetti, L., Perugi, G., Tundo, A., & Mignani, V. (1989). Psychopathology, temperament, and past course in primary major depressions: 1. Review of evidence for a bipolar spectrum. *Psychopathology, 22,* 268–277.

Akiskal, H. S., King, D., Rosenthal, T. L., Robinson, D., & Scott-Strauss, A. (1981). Chronic depressions, part 1: Clinical and familial characteristics. *Journal of Affective Disorders, 3,* 297–315.

Akiskal, H. S., & Mallya, G. D. (1987). Criteria for the "soft" bipolar spectrum. Treatment implications. *Psychopharmacologic Bulletin, 23,* 68–73.

American Psychiatric Association. (1987). *Diagnostic and statistical manual of mental disorders* (3rd ed., rev.). Washington, DC: Author.

Cassano, G. B., Akiskal, H. S., Musetti, L., Perugi, G., Soriani, A., & Mignani, V. (1989). Psychopathology, temperament, and past course in primary major depressions: 2. Toward a redefinition of bipolarity with a new semistructured interview for depression. *Psychopathology, 22,* 278–288.

Cassano, G. B., Akiskal, H. S., Perogi, G., Musetti, L., & Savino, M. (1992). The importance of measures of affective temperaments in genetic studies of mood disorders. *Journal of Psychiatric Research, 26*(4), 257–268.

Cassano, G. B., Maggini, C., & Akiskal, H. S. (1983). Short-term subchronic and chronic sequelae of affective disorders. *Psychiatric Clinics of North America, 6,* 55–68.

Cassano, G. B., & Savino, M. (1993). Chronic major depressive episode and dysthymia: Comparison of demographic and clinical characteristics. *European Psychiatry, 8,* 277–279.

Coryell, W., Endicott, J., Andreasen, N. C., Keller, M. B., Clayton, P. J. Hirschfeld, R. M. A., Scheftner, W. A., & Winokur, G. (1988). Depression and panic attacks: The significance of overlap as reflected in follow-up and family study data. *American Journal of Psychiatry, 145,* 293–300.

Derogatis, L. R., Lipman, R. S., & Rickel, S. K. (1973). The Hopkins Symptom Checklist (HSCL-90): A measure of primary symptom dimensions in psychological measurement. In P. Pichot (Ed.), *Modern problems in pharmacopsychiatry* (pp. 79–110). Basel: Karger.

Feinstein, A. R. (1970). The pre-therapeutic classification of co-morbidity in chronic disease. *Journal of Chronic Diseases, 23,* 445–468.

Hamilton, M. (1960). Development of a rating scale for primary depressive illness. *British Journal of Social Clinical Psychology, 6,* 178–196.

Hirschfeld, R. M. A., Klerman, G. L., Andreasen, N. C., Clayton, P. J., & Keller, M. B. (1986). Psycho-social predictors of chronicity in depressed patients. *British Journal of Psychiatry, 148,* 648–654.

Kerr, T. A., Roth, M., Schapira, K., & Gurney, C. (1972). The assessment and prediction of outcome in affective disorders. *British Journal of Psychiatry, 121,* 167–174.

Kraepelin, E. (1913). *Lectures on clinical psychiatry* (T. Johnstone, Ed.). London: Balliere, Tindall, & Cox.

Musetti, L., Perugi, G., Soriani, A., & Cassano, G. B. (1987). La depressione maggiore cronica: Indagine su 176 pazienti ambulatoriali. *Rivista di Psichiatria, 22,* 228–240.

Nystrom, S. (1979). Depression: Factors related to 10 years prognosis. *Acta Psychiatrica Scandinavica, 60,* 225–238.

Perugi, G., Maremmani, I., McNair, D. M., Cassano, G. B., & Akiskal, H. S. (1988). Differential changes in areas of social adjustment from depressive episodes through recovery. *Journal of Affective Disorders, 15,* 39–43.

Robins, E., & Guze, S. (1972). Classification of affective disorders: The primary-secondary, the endogenous and the neurotic–psychotic concepts. In T. A. Williams, M. M. Katz, & J. A. Shield (Eds.), *Recent advances in the psychobiology of depressive illness* (pp. 283–293). Washington, DC: U.S. Government Printing Office.

Savino, M., Perugi, G., Musetti, L., Soriani, A., Mignani, V., & Cassano, G. B. (1989). La depressione maggiore cronica: caratteristiche diagnostiche e cliniche. In G. C. Reda (Ed.), *Progressi in psichiatria* (Vol. 3, pp. 1401–1405). Roma: P. Pancheri.

Scott, J., Barker, W. A., & Eccleston, D. (1988). The Newcastle chronic depression study: Patient characteristics and factors associated with chronicity. *British Journal of Psychiatry, 152,* 28–33.

Scott, J. (1988). Chronic depression. *British Journal of Psychiatry, 153,* 287–297.

Van Valkenburg, C., Akiskal, H. S., Puzantian, V., & Rosenthal, T. (1984). Anxious depression: Clinical, family history, and naturalistic outcome—comparison with panic and major depressive disorders. *Journal of Affective Disorders, 6,* 67–82.

Weissman, M. M., Leaf, P. J., Bruce, M. L., & Florio, L. (1988). The epidemiology of dysthymia in five communities: Rates, risks, comorbidity and treatment. *American Journal of Psychiatry, 145,* 815–819.

CHAPTER 5

Chronic Depression: The Efficacy of Pharmacotherapy

James H. Kocsis

This chapter documents the efficacy of pharmacotherapy in chronic depressive illness irrespective of concurrent character pathology. It derives largely from the author's ongoing double-blind randomized trials of classical antidepressants.

The Nature of Chronic Depression

By the early 1980s we had become interested in studying the treatment of patients with chronic or "lifelong" states of depression. Our interest was stimulated by anecdotal clinical observations of dramatic response in several patients we treated with thymoleptic agents, as well as published reports of success in open clinical trials, principally those of Akiskal et al. (1980) and Ward et al. (1979).

These events prompted us to design a controlled clinical trial of imipramine versus placebo treatment for chronic depression (Kocsis et al., 1985, 1988a, 1988b). The publication of the DSM-III (American Psychiatric Association, 1980) criteria for dysthymic disorder provided a convenient basis for the definition of a sample for inclusion. We chose imipramine (IMI) because it was the standard antidepressant medication at the time in the United States. We hypothesized that no particular thymoleptic would be selectively indicated for the chronic depressives, and we wanted a generalizable result.

It quickly became apparent as we began to screen subjects that the threshold of symptom severity used to define major depressive disorder

(MDD) in DSM-III was very close to that of dysthymic disorder (DD). Thus, the chronic and lifelong depressives who presented to psychiatric clinics usually met the DSM-III criteria for both MDD and DD, a phenomenon which Keller and Shapiro (1982) termed "double depression."

Our clinical impression was that DD usually came on insidiously and would wax and wane in severity over time. Patients usually sought treatment during one of the more severe phases. We believed that the "superimposed" MDD represented a quantitative fluctuation in symptomatology of dysthymia, not a qualitatively different diagnostic entity. Eventually we proposed that double depression reflected an artifact of an inadequate nosological system for classifying mood disorders (Kocsis & Frances, 1987).

Based on these considerations we decided to include all chronic depressives who met criteria for DD in our studies, regardless of whether they also currently met the criteria for MDD.

A major issue that arose in the design of the studies was the definition of response. Our clinical observations of the course of dysthymia had been substantiated by the publication of a naturalistic follow-up of double depressives by Keller et al. (1983). This study found that patients with double depression frequently remitted partially to a state of dysthymia, then relapsed to a state of major depression during a 2-year period. Thus it seemed important to define response in these studies as a full and sustained remission from most or all depressive symptoms. Such criteria would be consistent with the definition of full remission from depression developed by a MacArthur Foundation network (Frank et al., 1991).

Another area of methodological difficulty became apparent during the conduct of these studies. Traditional scales for rating depressive symptom severity and change appeared to be somewhat inappropriate for outpatients with early onset DD because they had been developed for acute severe or psychotic episodes of major depression (e.g., the Hamilton Rating Scale for Depression [HAM-D]; Hamilton, 1960), or they were designed to rate acute symptoms based on comparison with normal recent premorbid states (e.g., the Beck Depression Inventory; Beck et al., 1961). These observations led us to the development of the Cornell Dysthymia Rating Scale (CDRS; Mason et al., 1993), a 20-item scale with good psychometric properties, which specifically focused on milder chronic symptoms of the type characteristic of patients with dysthymia.

The Short-Term Imipramine Study

This study was conducted in two psychiatric outpatient clinics located in New York and Maine (Kocsis et al., 1985, 1988a). In addition to a DSM-III diagnosis for DD, we required a 24-item HAM-D score greater than 13 for entry. Following a 2-week, single-blind placebo period, 54 patients were randomized to IMI (n = 29) or placebo (n = 25). All randomized subjects met the DSM-III criteria for both DD and MDD. Significantly more IMI patients (seven) than placebo (one) dropped out because of side effects. Remission was defined as a total score less than 7 on the HAM-D, a 10-point or greater increase in the Global Assessment Scale (GAS; Endicott et al., 1976) and no longer fulfilling the symptom criteria for DSM-III DD (based on CDRS rating scores). Forty-five percent of those randomized and 59% of those completing 6 weeks of IMI treatment (mean peak daily dose $\pm$ SD = 198 $\pm$ 59 mg/day) were remitted, compared to 13% of those completing placebo trials. Thus IMI appeared to be effective for short-term relief of depressive symptoms in chronic depressives meeting the DSM-III criteria for both DD and MDD at the time of treatment.

In the course of this study, we also became impressed by dramatic rapid improvement in social–vocational function in those patients who responded to IMI. In order to further document and study this phenomenon, we instituted the self-rated Social Adjustment Scale (SAS-SR; Weissman et al., 1978) before and after treatment. The IMI-treated subsample demonstrated marked and significant improvement over the 6-week period compared to the placebo group (Kocsis et al., 1988b). This finding was important. It suggested that many of the social–vocational impairments in patients with DD, which had given the disorder a "characterological" flavor, might indeed reflect chronic symptoms of a state of depression amenable to pharmacotherapy. We continued to pursue this issue in a long-term, naturalistic follow-up study of the IMI study participants (Kocsis et al., 1991). Nine IMI responders and an equal number of nonresponders were interviewed a mean of 40 months following entry into the study. Two-thirds of both groups were taking antidepressant medication at the time of assessment. The former IMI responder group was much better off than the nonresponders at the follow-up. Eight of the nine responders were still remitted. The responders scored significantly better on the HAM-D, GAS, and SAS-SR; of special note was that the mean SAS-SR score of 1.68 approached the reported normal score in community samples.

The results of the short-term IMI study and the long-term naturalistic follow-up study created a great deal of interest in the longer-term treatment of patients with chronic depression. We decided to make this our next research focus.

The Long-Term Desipramine Study

Our long-term desipramine (DMI) study consisted of three phases, similar to the design chosen for the National Institute of Mental Health

Collaborative Pharmacotherapy of Depression Study of Prien et al. (1984). *Acute treatment* was given for up to 10 weeks using open DMI in an attempt to suppress depressive symptoms. Study physicians could obtain plasma drug concentrations to optimize dosing. DMI was chosen for this study because of the high dropout rate seen with IMI in the previous study (24% over 6 weeks), which had mostly related to anticholinergic side effects. Responders to acute treatment then proceeded to *continuation treatment* for an additional 16 weeks for the purpose of stabilization and prevention of relapse. Responders could be subgrouped into those with full or partial remission. Full remission was defined as a 24-item HAM-D score less than 7 and a GAS score greater than 70 on three successive ratings over a 4-week period. Partial remission was defined as at least a 50% reduction from the baseline HAM-D score, HAM-D scores ranging from 7 to 12 and, GAS scores of 60 or greater over a 4-week period.

Subjects who met the criteria for either full or partial remission at the end of the continuation phase then were either randomized to *maintenance treatment* with continued DMI or tapered to placebo over a 1-month period. Both groups were followed and rated monthly for the next 2 years or until relapse. We hypothesized that maintenance treatment with DMI would lead to a lower rate of relapse among patients with DD who had responded favorably to acute and continuation treatment. *Relapse* was defined as a period of 4 or more weeks with HAM-D scores above 12 and meeting the DSM-III-R (American Psychiatric Association, 1987) symptom criteria for dysthymia, *or* at least one rating meeting these criteria plus an urgent need for alternative treatment for depression. Results have now been reported (Kocsis et al., 1996): Four of the 27 DMI (15%) and 12/23 (52%) placebo patients relapsed during the maintenance phase, a highly significant difference. From a clinical perspective, then, discontinuation of active medication, even after a prolonged period of stabilization of remission, was associated with a substantial risk of relapse in these chronic depressions.

A number of subsidiary clinical questions are also being addressed by this long-term study. Using newspaper advertising we were able to increase the proportion of subjects with "pure" dysthymia (e.g., not currently meeting criteria for MDD. Thus, of the 129 cases entering the long-term study, 60% did and 40% did not fulfill criteria for MDD. Rates of remission during the acute phase were higher, although not significantly so, for the pure dysthymia (57%) than for the double depression (47%) subgroup. Proportions of full to partial remission were approximately 2:1 in both groups. These results created equal sized groups of pure dysthymia and double-depression randomized to active DMI or placebo in the maintenance phase. However, this diagnostic distinction did not appear to affect the relapse rates. Both groups experienced high relapse rates on placebo and low rates on active drug. This result suggested that both short- and longer-term treatment may be indicated and effective for both diagnostic subgroups of chronic depression.

Another question we addressed was whether full versus partial remission would predict the outcome of the maintenance treatment with either the continued active DMI or the placebo. We reported data on 40 full and 10 partially remitted cases in the maintenance phase. Two of five partial and 10/18 full remitters relapsed on placebo. Thus, even a prolonged period of full remission from depressive symptoms did not appear to have produced "recovery" in the majority of these chronic depressives. It appears that many patients may require continued long-term treatment to suppress the depressive symptomatology and to facilitate social–vocational rehabilitation.

Studies of Comorbidity of Dysthymia

Akiskal (1983) proposed subtyping dysthymia. A number of the criteria proposed related to comorbidity with anxiety or personality disorders. When we began our clinical studies, we hypothesized that dysthymia would be associated with a high prevalence of Axis II diagnoses, especially borderline personality disorder, and that Axis II diagnoses would predict poor response to antidepressant medication. Subsequently we conducted three studies of dysthymia's comorbidity. Markowitz et al. (1992) interviewed 75 consecutive psychiatric outpatients using the Structured Clinical Interview for DSM-III-R (SCID; Spitzer & Williams, 1985; Spitzer et al., 1986) for both Axis I and Axis II. Thirty-six percent of the sample met the DSM-III-R criteria for dysthymia. Dysthymic outpatients (n = 34) were significantly more likely than the comparison (nondysthymic) group to meet the criteria for major depression (68%), social phobia (15%), avoidant (32%), self-defeating (35%), dependent (21%), and borderline (24%) personality disorders. Eighty-five percent of the sample was found to have an Axis II diagnosis using the SCID-II method of diagnosis, and 56% met criteria for two or more. Treatment implications were not addressed in this study.

In a second study, Marin et al. (1993) assessed 49 patients with dysthymia and 19 patients with episodic major depression using the Personality Disorder Examination (PDE; Loranger et al., 1987). This is a more stringent method of Axis II diagnosis and lower prevalences were found. Fifty-one percent of the dysthymia, and 42% of the episodic major depression group met criteria for a personality disorder. The most highly prevalent diagnoses in the dysthymia group were personality disorder not otherwise specified (22%), avoidant (20%), and dependent (8%). Only three patients (6%) had a borderline personality. Episodic major depression had similar rates and patterns of personality diagnosis. We subsequently examined the effect of an Axis II diagnosis on the outcome of treatment during the acute phase of the DMI study described above. Fifty-nine patients with dysthymia who entered the DMI trial of open treatment were given the PDE interview. Thirty-one (53%) had an Axis II diagnosis. The treatment outcomes are shown in Table 5.1.

A comorbid Axis II diagnosis had no effect on outcome in this sample. Of patients completing treatment, 50% with and 38% with no Axis II diagnosis achieved full remission.

The third study by Lewinter et al. (1993) addressed the implications of a comorbid anxiety disorder. Eighty-two subjects entering the DMI study received the SCID-I interview. Nineteen of these (23%) met criteria for an anxiety disorder, with the most prevalent diagnosis being generalized anxiety disorder (15%) and social phobia (8%). Treatment outcomes are shown in Table 5.2.

Again, there is no apparent effect of the comorbidity on the treatment outcome. Among those patients completing the treatment, 32% with and 33% without an anxiety disorder achieved full remission.

TABLE 5.1. Response to Open DMI with or without an Axis II Diagnosis

Outcome	Axis II	No Axis II	Total
Full remission	13	8	21
Partial remission	7	5	12
Nonresponder	6	8	14
Dropout	5	7	12
Total	31	28	59

TABLE 5.2. Response to Open DMI with or without an Anxiety Disorder

Outcome	Anxiety disorder	No anxiety disorder	Total
Full remission	6	21	27
Partial remission	1	13	14
Nonresponder	6	16	22
Dropout	6	13	19
Total	19	63	82

Conclusions

We believe these have been the first placebo-controlled clinical trials of short- and long-term use of tricyclic antidepressants in outpatients selected for chronic depression using the DSM-III criteria. Along with other studies reported in this volume, the short-term efficacy of a number of classes of thymoleptic medication has now been established for these patients. The question of the utility and the value of longer-term treatment will require further research, but it does appear to be promising. Although about 50% of patients with dysthymia appear to respond very favorably to antidepressant medications, the issue of subtyping with predictive validity for treatment response has remained elusive in our hands (Kocsis et al., 1989).

Contrary to clinical lore, concurrent personality disorders do not seem to diminish the likelihood of positive responses to pharmacotherapy. The implication of our studies for the clinician are clear: Irrespective of Axis II diagnoses, all chronic depressives should be seriously considered for pharmacotherapy. Should the first agent fail, sequential adequate empirical trials using the major classes of antidepressants appear merited in the treatment of chronic depression.

References

Akiskal, H. S. (1983). Dysthymic disorder: Psychopathology of proposed chronic depressive subtypes. *American Journal of Psychiatry, 140*, 11–20.

Akiskal, H. S., Rosenthal, T. L., Haykal, R. F., Lemmi, H., Rosethal, R. H., & Scott-Straus, A. (1980). Characterologic depressions. *Archives of General Psychiatry, 37*, 777–783.

American Psychiatric Association. (1980). *Diagnostic and statistical manual of mental disorders* (3rd ed.). Washington, DC: Author.

American Psychiatric Association. (1987). *Diagnostic and statistical manual of mental disorders* (3rd ed., rev.). Washington, DC: Author.

Beck, A., Ward, C., Mendelson, H., Mock, D., & Erbaugh, J. (1961). An inventory for measuring depression. *Archives of General Psychiatry, 4*, 53–63.

Endicott, J., Spitzer, R. L., Fleiss, J. L., Cohen, J. (1976). The global assessment scale: A procedure for measuring the overall severity of psychiatric disturbance. *Archives of General Psychiatry, 33*, 767–771.

Frank, E., Prien, R. F., Jarrett, R. B., Keller, M. B., Kupfer, D. J., Lavori, P. W., Rush, A. J., & Weissman, M. M. (1991). Conceptualization and rationale for consensus definitions of terms in major depressive disorders: Remission, relapse, recovery, recurrence. *Archives of General Psychiatry, 48*, 851–855.

Hamilton, M. (1960). Rating scale for depression. *Journal of Neurology and Neurosurgical Psychiatry, 25*, 56–62.

Keller, M. B., Lavori, P. W., Endicott, J., Coryell, W., & Klerman, G. L. (1983). "Double depression": Two-year follow-up. *American Journal of Psychiatry, 140,* 689–694.

Keller, M. B., & Shapiro, R. W. (1982). "Double depression": Superimposition of acute depressive episodes on chronic depressive disorders. *American Journal of Psychiatry, 139,* 438–442.

Kocsis, J. H., & Frances, A. J. (1987). A critical discussion of DSM-III dysthymic disorder. *American Journal of Psychiatry, 144,* 1534–1542.

Kocsis, J. H., Frances A. J., Mann, J. J., Sweeney, J., Voss, C., Mason, B., & Brown, R. P. (1985). Imipramine for the treatment of chronic depression. *Psychopharmacology Bulletin, 21,* 698–700.

Kocsis, J. H., Frances, A. J., Voss, C., Mann, J. J., Mason, B. J., & Sweeney, J. (1988a). Imipramine treatment for chronic depression. *Archives of General Psychiatry, 45,* 253–257.

Kocsis, J. H., Frances, A. J., Voss, C., Mason, B. J., & Mann, J. J. (1988b). Effects of imipramine treatment on social–vocational adjustment in chronic depression. *American Journal of Psychiatry, 145,* 997–999.

Kocsis, J. H., Friedman, R. A., Markowitz, J. C., Leon, A. C., Miller, N. L., Gniewesch, L., & Parides, M. (1996). Maintenance therapy for chronic depression: A controlled clinical trial of desipramine. *Archives of General Psychiatry, 53,* 769–774.

Kocsis, J. H., Mason, B. J., Frances, A. J., Sweeney, J., Mann, J. J., & Marin, D. (1989). Prediction of response of chronic depression to imipramine. *Journal of Affective Disorders, 17,* 255–260.

Kocsis, J. H., Sutton, B. M., & Frances, A. J. (1991). Long-term follow-up of chronic depression treated with imipramine. *Journal of Clinical Psychiatry, 52,* 56–59.

Lewinter, D., Kocsis, J. H., & Markowitz, J. C. (1993). *Impact of comorbid anxiety on antidepressant response in dysthymia.* Unpublished manuscript, Cornell University Medical College, New York.

Loranger, A., Susman, V., Oldham, J., & Russakoff, L. M. (1987). The personality disorder examination: A preliminary report. *Journal of Personality Disorders, 1,* 1–13.

Marin, D. B., Kocsis, J. H., Frances, A. J., & Klerman, G. L. (1993). Personality disorders in dysthymia. *Journal of Personality Disorders, 7,* 223–631.

Markowitz, J. C., Moran, M. E., Kocsis, J. H., & Frances, A. J. (1992). Prevalence and comorbidity of dysthymic disorder among psychiatric outpatients. *Journal of Affective Disorders, 24,* 63–71.

Mason, B. J., Kocsis, J. H., Leon, A. C., Frances, A. J., Morgan, R. O., Parides, M. K., & Thompson, S. (1993). Measurement of severity and treatment response in dysthymia. *Psychiatric Annals, 23,* 625–631.

Prien, R. F., Kupfer, D. J., Mansky, P. A., Small, J. G., Tuason, V. B., Voss, C. B., & Johnson, W. E. (1984). Drug therapy in the prevention of recurrences in unipolar and bipolar affective disorders. *Archives of General Psychiatry, 41,* 1096–1104.

Spitzer, R. L., & Williams, J. B. W. (1985). *Structured Clinical Interview for DSM-III-Patient version (SCID-P, 3/1/85)*. New York: Biometrics Research Department, New York State Psychiatric Institute.

Spitzer, R. L., Williams, J. B. W., & Gibbon, M. (1986). *Structured Clinical Interview for DSM-III-R Personality Disorders (SCID-II, 10/15/86)*. New York: Biometrics Research Department, New York State Psychiatric Institute.

Ward, N. G., Bloom, V. L., & Friedel, R. O. (1979). The effectiveness of tricyclic antidepressants in chronic depression. *Journal of Clinical Psychiatry, 40,* 49–52.

Weissman, M. M., Prusoff, B. A., Thompson, W. D., Harding, P. S., & Myers, J. K. (1978). Social adjustment by self-report in a community sample and in psychiatric outpatients. *Journal of Nervous and Mental Disease, 166,* 317–326.

CHAPTER 6

"Residual States" in Affective, Schizoaffective, and Schizophrenic Disorders

Andreas Marneros
Anke Rohde

Recent research clearly indicates that not only schizophrenic and schizoaffective disorders but also affective disorders can leave persistent psychopathological and psychosocial alterations (Angst, 1980, 1986, 1987; Berti Ceroni et al., 1984; Deister et al., 1990; Goodwin & Jamison, 1990; Marneros et al., 1990, 1991; Mueller & Leon, 1996; van Os et al., 1996). The phenomenology of persistent alterations in schizophrenia has been described repeatedly, sometimes extensively, especially by German psychopathologists (Huber et al., 1979; Janzarik, 1968; Mundt, 1985). In contrast, the research regarding persistent alterations in affective disorders is limited to the evaluation of the frequency and global type of the so-called chronic depression (Marneros & Deister, 1990; Marneros et al., 1991), and practically no research has been carried out on the phenomenology of persistent alterations in schizoaffective disorders. Similarly, research comparing the phenomenology of all three functional psychotic disorders is nonexistent.

Modern descriptions of phenomenological aspects of persistent alterations ("residual states") in affective, schizoaffective, and schizophrenic disorders often reflect simply items, scores, and variables of scales and evaluation instruments. But the operational structure and intention of such instruments have a limiting or even an inhibiting impact on the phenomenological picture. It is difficult to describe phenomenological constellations of persistent alterations in functional psychotic disorders, mainly because of the high degree of individuality and changeability of patterns of course and elements of phenomenology (Janzarik, 1968; Mundt, 1985; Marneros et al. 1991). In spite of such difficulties and limitations, however, many reports of long-term research have described "residual types" of schizophrenic as well as affective disorders (e.g., Bleuler, 1972; Huber et al., 1979; Ciompi & Muller, 1976; see also overviews in Goodwin & Jamison 1990; Marneros et al., 1991). However, it is difficult to consider the full richness and variability of phenomenological constellations of persistent alterations. If we nevertheless attempt to consider the richness, variability, changeability, and individuality of phenomenological and interactional aspects, it is nearly impossible to paint a picture that has general validity; instead, we merely collect individual profiles. The fine psychopathological descriptions by Huber et al. (1979) in Germany delineated 15 different types of residual states for schizophrenic patients alone. However, most of these 15 types had a frequency of 0.4% to 9%. If we try to describe only global categories of residual states—as, for instance, M. Bleuler (1972) did—the groups described are phenomenologically extremely heterogeneous. If we try to describe residual states only according to the various operational criteria, it is possible that important aspects such as clinical impressions, clinical atmosphere, and the interactions between patients and their social environment will be lost.

Therefore, this chapter attempts to integrate operationally gathered findings with clinical and interactional aspects, resulting in phenomenological constellations of persistent alterations applicable to all groups of functional psychotic disorders. The description of the presented syndromes of persistent alterations is atheoretical, without any ambitions regarding psychodynamic interpretations or etiopathological assumptions.

Design of Study and Description of Patients

This study forms part of the Cologne study on the long-term course and outcome of patients with functional psychotic disorders (Marneros et al., 1988, 1989, 1990, 1991). The psychopathological, psychological, and social status of 402 patients was evaluated during a mean observation period of more than 25 years (see Table 6.1). One hundred and forty-eight patients were diagnosed longitudinally according to slightly modified DSM-III (American Psychiatric Association, 1980) criteria as having schizophrenia,

TABLE 6.1. Study Population

	Schizophrenic disorders	Schizoaffective disorders	Affective disorders
Number of patients	148	101	106
Sex distribution			
Male	86 (58.1%)	37 (36.6%)	26 (24.5%)
Female	62 (41.9%)	64 (63.4%)	80 (75.5%)
Age at onset (years)			
Arithmetic mean	27.7	30.4	36.1
Median	24.0	29.0	35.0
SD	10.6	10.4	11.0
Range	14–64	15–58	15–63
Length of observation time			
Arithmetic mean	23.0	25.5	27.9
Median	25.0	25.0	25.0
SD	9.9	10.5	9.3
Range	10–50	10–61	10–56
Age at end of observation time			
Arithmetic mean	50.7	55.9	64.0
Median	51.0	54.0	66.0
SD	13.2	14.0	12.5
Range	27–84	27–87	32–87

101 as having schizoaffective disorder, and 106 as having affective disorders.

All recorded episodes during the course were evaluated and defined according to slightly modified DSM-III criteria (see Marneros et al. 1988, 1991, for a detailed description of the criteria for episodes). In summary:

- A *schizophrenic disorder* was diagnosed if only schizophrenic episodes occurred during the whole observation period with no affective and no schizoaffective episodes.
- An *affective disorder* was diagnosed if only affective (melancholic, manic, or manic–depressive mixed) episodes were found, with no schizophrenic or schizoaffective (schizomanic, schizodepressive, or schizomanic–depressive mixed) episodes occurring during course.
- The diagnosis *schizoaffective disorder* was made if (1) schizoaffective (schizomanic, schizodepressive, or schizomanic–depressive mixed) episodes were present at least once during the course, or (2) both schizophrenic and affective (manic, melancholic, or manic–depressive mixed) episodes occurred, regardless of their number, sequence, or relative frequency.

In the first methodological stage we interviewed personally and examined all the patients using the following instruments to evaluate their psychopathological and psychosocial status at the end of the observation period:

- Present State Examination (PSE; Wing et al., 1974)
- Modified version of PSE for follow-up
- Global Assessment Scale (GAS; Spitzer et al., 1976)
- Disability Assessment Schedule (WHO/DAS; World Health Organization, 1988)
- Psychological Impairments Rating Schedule (WHO/PIRS; Biehl et al.,1989)
- General sociodemographic schedule based mainly on items of
  - Psychiatric and Personal History Schedule (PPHS; World Health Organization, 1985c)
  - Follow-Up History and Sociodemographic Description Schedule (FU-HSD; World Health Organization, 1985a)
- Past History and Sociodemographic Description Schedule (PHSD; World Health Organization, 1985b)
- Own items of social consequences of the illness:
  - Social mobility
  - Occupational mobility
  - Premature retirement
  - "Achievement of the expected social development"
  - Autarky (living situation at the end of the observation time)

Persistent alterations were defined as the persistence of deficits, impairments, and alterations in the domains of psychopathology and psychological and social functions for more than 3 years (Marneros et al., 1989).

To obtain the most complex clinical and interactional impression of the patient and the clearest picture of the degree and type of persistent alterations, we recorded the interview with the patient and the family members present on audiotape. In addition, the interviewer made a protocol of his global impression of the patient and the interview situation, communication, and interaction with the patient and other interesting observations. The tapes were then evaluated once again separately, taking into account all other available information and the results of the several standardized instruments applied, to evaluate the outcome.

Cluster analysis methods proved to be insufficient to reflect the true status. As we mentioned earlier, the consideration of only operationally defined items ignores a great part of the clinical impressions and of the "interactional atmosphere" between patients and their environment. For this reason we renounced cluster analysis in favor of a *descriptive case analysis,* creating an individual *phenomenological profile* for every patient. This profile was based on the following:

- Results from the PSE
- Disturbed items of the WHO/PIRS
- Disturbances evaluated using the criteria of psychopathological "outcome" by Huber et al. (1979)
- The opinion of the clinician based on the clinical impression and the observed "interactional atmosphere"

In a further stage the phenomenological profiles were drawn up on five dimensions according to the "present/not present" principle (A = productive psychotic symptoms, B = loss of energy, C = quantitative changes in affectivity, D = qualitative changes in affectivity, and E = disturbances of behavior). A sixth dimension, "cognitive disturbances," proved to be strongly dependent on the other investigated dimensions and was not included.

The procedure described resulted in various phenomenological constellations of persistent alterations which could be classified into eight groups (for definitions see Table 6.2):

1. Depletion syndrome
2. Apathetic–paranoid syndrome (or apathetic–hallucinatory syndrome)
3. Adynamic deficiency syndrome
4. Chronic psychosis
5. Structural deformation of personality
6. Slight asthenic insufficiency syndrome
7. Chronic subdepressive syndrome
8. Chronic hyperthymic syndrome

Persistent Alterations

Persistent alterations—of varying degree and varying phenomenological constellation—were found in 93.2% (138) of the schizophrenic patients, in 49.5% of the patients with schizoaffective disorders, and in 35.8% of those with affective disorders. The persistent alterations began on average 1.6 years, 6.7 years, and 9.9 years after onset, respectively. Persistent alterations could manifest themselves at any time during the course. All three diagnostic groups included some patients who showed persistent alterations

TABLE 6.2. Phenomenological Constellations of Persistent Alterations

Depletion syndrome
  Severe reduction of drive
  Severe deficiency of energy and initiative
  Affective flattening
  Reduction of facial expressions and gestures
  "Cool isolation"
  Severe reduction of concentration capacity
  Increased distractibility
  Patients are not aware of their disturbances
  No persistent productive psychotic symptoms

Apathetic–paranoid syndrome (or apathetic–hallucinatory syndrome)
  Persistent delusions and/or hallucinations
  Severe slowness
  Affective flattening
  Severe social withdrawal
  Loss of interest for almost all activities
  Severe reduction of energy and initiative
  Patients are not aware of their disturbances

Adynamic deficiency syndrome
  Moderate reduction of the mental energetic potential
  Reduction of interest for everyday events
  Affectivity reduced, but not flattened
  Limited variation of behavior and expression
  No "cool isolation"
  No continuous depressive or euphoric mood
  Productive psychotic symptoms only transient and not impressive

Chronic psychosis
  Chronic productive psychotic symptomatology (in most cases paranoid
    symptomatology)
  No severe disturbances of affectivity, possibly slight fluctuations of mood
  No severe disturbances of expression and contact

Structural deformation of personality
  Persistent deformation of the personality
  Productive psychotic symptoms only transient and not impressive
  No severe disturbances of affectivity
  No slowness

Slight asthenic insufficiency syndrome
  Slight reduction of mental energetic potential
  Possibly slight, subjective perceived impairments of concentration capacity
  Slight mood disturbances
  No productive psychotic symptoms or only transient and not impressive

Chronic subdepressive syndrome
  Chronic subdepressive symptoms
  No affective flattening
  No productive psychotic symptomatology
  No slowness

Chronic hyperthymic syndrome
  Chronic hyperthymic symptomatology
  No affective flattening
  No productive psychotic symptomatology
  No slowness

directly after onset and others who first displayed such alterations 20 or even 30 years after onset.

Comparison of the mean values of GAS total scores showed significant differences between the three groups. The affective disorders had the most favorable outcome, with a mean score of 87.4, and schizophrenic disorders had the worst, with a mean score of 42.1. Schizoaffective disorders occupied an intermediate position with a mean score of 76.2, closer to the affective than to the schizophrenic disorders (Table 6.3).

Similar differences were found among the three groups when the disability was assessed using WHO/DAS (World Health Organization, 1988) and WHO/PIRS (Marneros et al., 1989, 1990, 1991).

Significant differences among the three diagnostic groups were also found with regard to social consequences of the illness after long-term course, especially between schizophrenic disorders on the one hand and schizoaffective and affective disorders on the other. The differences between affective and schizoaffective disorders regarding social consequences are mainly nonsignificant (Table 6.3). *Negative social consequences* of the illness were significantly more frequent in schizophrenic than in schizoaffective or affective disorders, whereas no differences were found between affective and schizoaffective patients (Table 6.3).

Distribution of Various Types of Phenomenological Constellations

Among the schizophrenic patients, the most frequently found phenomenological constellation was the apathetic–paranoid syndrome (or apathetic–hallucinatory syndrome), followed by the depletion syndrome and the adynamic deficiency syndrome. No cases of chronic subdepressive syndrome or chronic hyperthymic syndrome were found in schizophrenic patients. Among the schizoaffective disorders, the most frequent constellation was the asthenic insufficiency syndrome, followed by the adynamic deficiency syndrome. Depletion syndrome and chronic psychosis were not found in the schizoaffective disorders. Among the affective disorders, the most common syndrome was again the asthenic insufficiency syndrome, followed this time by the chronic subdepressive syndrome. Depletion syndrome, apathetic–paranoid syndrome, adynamic deficiency syndrome, chronic psychosis, and structural deformation did not occur in the affective disorders (Table 6.4).

Thus the persistent alterations in schizophrenia were clustered in the first six of the eight types of phenomenological constellations listed earlier and in affective disorders in the last three types, whereas in schizoaffective disorders they are distributed over the whole spectrum with the exception of the depletion syndrome and chronic psychosis.

TABLE 6.3. Aspects of Long-Term Outcome

	Schizophrenic disorders ($n = 148$)	S1	Schizoaffective disorders ($n = 101$)	S2	Affective disorders ($n = 106$)	S3
GAS		**		**		**
No disturbances (score 91–100)	10 (6.8%)		51 (50.5%)		68 (64.2%)	
Slight disturbances (score 71–90)	18 (12.2%)		14 (13.9%)		19 (17.9%)	
Moderate disturbances (score 51–70)	17 (11.5%)		15 (14.9%)		15 (14.2%)	
Severe disturbances (score 31–50)	28 (18.9%)		15 (14.9%)		4 (3.8%)	
Very severe disturbances (score 1–30)	75 (50.7%)		6 (5.9%)		–	
Arithmetic mean	42.1	**	76.2	**	87.4	**(2)
Median	30.0	**	91.0	*	95.0	**(3)
Standard deviation	26.1		26.8		15.6	
WHO/DAS (global evaluation)		**		**		**(1)
Excellent adjustment (score 0)	11 (7.4%)		55 (54.5%)		68 (64.2%)	
Very good adjustment (score 1)	13 (8.8%)		16 (15.8%)		21 (19.8%)	
Good adjustment (score 2)	29 (19.6%)		20 (19.8%)		8 (7.5%)	
Fair adjustment (score 3)	30 (20.3%)		1 (1.0%)		7 (6.6%)	
Poor adjustment (score 4)	40 (27.0%)		9 (8.9%)		2 (1.9%)	
Very poor adjustment (score 5)	25 (16.9%)		–		–	
Arithmetic mean	3.01	**	0.94	**	0.62	**(2)
Median	3.00	**	0.00	**	0.00	**(3)
Standard deviation	1.48		1.26		1.01	
Downward occupational drift	($n = 126$) 90 (71.4%)	**	($n = 69$) 29 (42.0%)	–	($n = 55$) 16 (29.1%)	**(1)
Downward social drift	($n = 90$) 63 (70.0%)	**	($n = 65$) 15 (23.1%)	–	($n = 45$) 11 (24.%)	**(1)
Premature retirement (because of mental illness)	($n = 125$) 63 (50.4%)	**	($n = 69$) 18 (26.1%)	–	($n = 55$) 14 (25.5%)	**(1)
Achievement of the expected social development	($n = 148$) 45 (30.4%)	**	($n = 101$) 72 (71.3%)	–	($n = 106$) 87 (82.1%)	**(1)
Impairment of autarky (because of mental illness)	($n = 144$) 85 (59.0%)	**	($n = 91$) 20 (22.0%)	*	($n = 83$) 6 (7.2%)	**(1)

Note. Significance: S1, schizophrenic disorders versus schizoaffective disorders; S2, schizoaffective disorders versus affective disorders; S3, affective disorders versus schizophrenic disorders. (1) χ^2 test; (2) t test; (3) Mann–Whitney U test

*$p < .05$.

**$p = .01$.

TABLE 6.4. Frequency of Phenomenological Alterations (Patients with Persistent Alterations)

	Schizophrenic disorders (n = 138)	Schizoaffective disorders (n = 50)	Affective disorders (n = 38)
Depletion syndrome	31 (20.9%)	—	—
Apathetic–paranoid syndrome (or apathetic–hallucinatory syndrome)	51 (34.5%)	5 (5.0%)	—
Adynamic deficiency syndrome	30 (20.3%)	16 (15.8%)	—
Chronic psychosis	10 (6.8%)	—	—
Structural deformation of personality structure	5 (3.4%)	2 (2.0%)	—
Slight asthenic insufficiency syndrome	11 (7.4%)	19 (18.8%)	22 (20.8%)
Chronic subdepressive syndrome	—	4 (4.0%)	14 (13.2%)
Chronic hyperthymic syndrome	—	4 (4.0%)	2 (1.9%)

Discussion and Conclusions

Investigating the long-term outcome of affective, schizoaffective, and schizophrenic disorders, persistent alterations ("residual states") were found in all three groups. A high proportion (93%) of schizophrenic patients had persistent alterations in several aspects of social life, communication, and cognitive functions, in some cases to a high degree. Although the outcome of affective disorders is not always favorable (persistent alterations in 35.8% of cases), overall it is significantly more favorable than that of schizophrenia. Schizoaffective disorders occupy an intermediate position regarding outcome (49.5% persistent alterations), but closer to affective than to schizophrenic disorders.

Applying a model that integrated the operationally gathered findings (using WHO/DAS, WHO/PIRS, GAS, etc.) with the "interactional atmosphere" experienced by the clinician during the personal interaction with the patient and using the "clinical impression" as a connection between the instrumental findings, eight different types of phenomenological constellations of persistent alterations were delineated: (1) depletion syndrome, (2) apathetic–paranoid (or apathetic–hallucinatory) syndrome, (3) adynamic deficiency syndrome, (4) chronic psychosis, (5) structural deformation, (6) slight asthenic insufficiency syndrome, (7) chronic subdepressive syndrome, and (8) chronic hyperthymic syndrome. The advantage of this model is that it is applicable to all types of functional psychotic disorders, with the possibility of comparing the different groups. The description of the presented syndromes of persistent alterations is atheoretical, with no ambitions regarding interpretations or etiopathological considerations.

Only the slight asthenic insufficiency syndrome was found in all three investigated groups. The most frequent types in schizophrenic disorders were depletion syndrome (20.9%), apathetic–paranoid (or apathetic–hallucinatory) syndrome (34.5%), and adynamic deficiency syndrome (20.3%). Only three types of phenomenological constellations occurred in affective disorders: slight asthenic insufficiency syndrome (20.8%), chronic subdepressive syndrome (13.2%), and chronic hyperthymic syndrome (1.9%). As in the frequency of persistent alterations, schizoaffective disorders again held an intermediate position, featuring six of the eight types of phenomenological constellations (except depletion syndrome and chronic psychosis).

Former assumptions that cross-sectionally the persistent alterations in schizophrenia are usually indistinguishable from those in affective disorders could not be confirmed. Only 7% of the schizophrenic patients had persistent alterations that were phenomenologically similar to those in affective disorders. These differences in the phenomenology of persistent alterations between schizophrenic and affective disorders could perhaps be interpreted as a result of different biological and psychological processes. Schizoaffective disorders develop persistent alterations that are phenomenologically common to both affective and schizophrenic disorders, which might reflect the intermediate position held by schizoaffective disorders in many other regards, for instance, sociodemographic, premorbid variables, and parameters of long-term outcome.

Acknowledgment

We are grateful to Arno Deister, from the Psychiatric Hospital of the University of Bonn, for his participation in the research reported in this chapter.

References

American Psychiatric Association. (1980). *Diagnostic and statistical manual of mental disorders* (3rd ed.). Washington, DC: Author.
Angst, J. (1980). Verlauf Unipolar Depressiver, Bipolar Manischdepressiver und Schizo-affektiver Erkrankungen und Psychosen: Ergebnisse Einer Prospektiven Studie. *Fortschritte der Neurologie–Psychiatrie, 48,* 3–30.

Angst, J. (1986). The course of schizoaffective disorders. In A. Marneros & M. T. Tsuang (Eds.), *Schizoaffective psychoses*. Berlin: Springer.

Angst. J. (1987). Verlauf der affektiven Psychosen. In K. P. Kisker, H. Lauter, J. E. Meyer, C. Muller, & E. Stromgren (Eds.), *Psychiatrie der Gegenwart* (Vol. 5). Berlin: Springer.

Berti Ceroni, G. B., Neri, C., & Pezzoli, A. (1984). Chronicity in major depression. A naturalistic prospective study. *Journal of Affective Disorders, 7*, 1224–1232.

Biehl, H., Maurer, K., Jablensky, A., Cooper, J. E., & Tomov, T. (1989). The WHO Psychological Impairments Rating Schedule (WHO/PIRS): I. Introducing a new instrument for rating observed behaviour and the rationale of the psychological impairment concept. *British Journal of Psychiatry, 155* (Suppl. 7), 68–70.

Bleuler, M. (1972). *Die schizophrenen Geistesstörungen im Lichte langjähriger Kranken- und Familiengeschichten*. Stuttgart: Thieme.

Ciompi, L., & Muller, C. (1976). *Lebensweg und Alter der Schizophrenen. Eine katamnestische Studie bis ins Senium*. Berlin: Springer.

Deister, A., Marneros, A., & Rohde, A. (1990). Long-term outcome of affective, schizoaffective and schizophrenic disorders: A comparison. In A. Marneros & M. T. Tsuang (Eds.), *Affective and schizoaffective disorders: Similarities and differences*. Berlin: Springer.

Glatzel, J., & Lungershausen, E. (1968). Zur Frage der Residualsyndrome nach thymoleptisch behandelten cyclothymen Depressionen. *Archiv für Psychiatrie Zeitschrift Gesamte Neurologie, 210*, 437–446.

Goodwin, F. K., & Jamison, K. R. (1990). *Manic–depressive illness*. New York: Oxford University Press.

Huber, G., Glatzel, J., & Lungershausen, E. (1969). Über zyklothyme Residualsyndrome. In W. Schulte & W. Mende (Eds.), *Melancholie in Forschung, Klinik und Behandlung*. Stuttgart: Thieme.

Huber, G., Gross, G., & Schüttler, R. (1979). *Schizophrenie. Eine verlaufs- und Sozialpsychiatrische Langzeitstudie*. Berlin: Springer.

Janzarik, W. (1968). *Schizophrene Verläufe: Eine Strukturdynamische Interpretation*. Berlin: Springer.

Marneros, A., & Deister, A. (1990). Chronische Depression. Psychopathologie, Verlaufsaspekte und Prädisponierende Faktoren. In H. J. Möller (Ed.), *Therapieresistenz unter Antidepressiva-Behandlung*. Berlin: Springer.

Marneros, A., Deister, A., & Rohde, A. (1990). Psychopathological and social status of patients with affective, schizophrenic and schizoaffective disorders after long-term course. *Acta Psychiatrica Scandinavica, 82*, 352–358.

Marneros, A., Deister, A., & Rohde, A. (1991). *Affektive, Schizoaffektive und Schizophrene Psychosen. Eine Vergleichende Langzeitstudie* [with detailed English summary]. Berlin: Springer.

Marneros, A., Deister, A., Rohde, A., Jünemann, H., & Fimmers, R. (1988). Long-term course of schizoaffective disorders: Part I. Definitions, methods, frequency of episodes and cycles. *European Archives of Psychiatry and Neurological Sciences, 237*, 264–275.

Marneros, A., Deister, A., Rohde, A., Steinmeyer, E. M., & Jünemann, H. (1989). Long-term outcome of schizoaffective and schizophrenic disorders: A comparative study: Part I. Definitions, methods, psychopathological and social outcome. *European Archives of Psychiatry and Neurological Sciences, 238,* 118–125.

Mueller, T. I. & Leon, A. C. (1996) Recovery, chronicity, and levels of psychopathology in major depression. *Psychiatry Clinics of North America, 19,* 85–102.

Mundt, C. (1985). *Das Apathiesyndrom der Schizophrenen: Eine Psychopathologische und Computertomographische Untersuchung.* Berlin: Springer.

Spitzer, R. L., Gibbon, M., & Endicott, J. (1976). The Global Assessment Scale. *Archives of General Psychiatry, 33,* 768–773.

van Os, J., Fahy, T. A., Jones, P., Harvey, I., Sham, P., Lewis, S., Bebbington, P., Toone, B., Williams, M., & Murray, R. (1996). Psychopathological syndromes in the functional psychoses: Associations with course and outcome. *Psychological Medicine, 26,* 161–176.

Wing, J. K., Cooper, J. E., & Sartorius, N. (1974). *Measurement and classification of psychiatric symptoms.* Cambridge, UK: Cambridge University Press.

World Health Organization. (1985a). *Follow-up History and Sociodemographic Description Schedule (FU-HSD).* Geneva: Author.

World Health Organization. (1985b). *Past History and Sociodemographic Description Schedule (PHSD).* Geneva: Author.

World Health Organization. (1985c). *Psychiatric and Personal History Schedule (PPHS).* Geneva: Author.

World Health Organization. (1988). *WHO Psychiatric Disability Assessment Schedule (WHO/DAS).* Geneva: Author.

CHAPTER 7

Depressive Personality: Relationship to Dysthymia and Major Depression

Daniel N. Klein
Gregory A. Miller

The concept of the depressive personality has been widely used in the clinical literature, particularly in the works of psychodynamic and descriptive-phenomenological authors (Kernberg, 1988; Phillips et al., 1990; Akiskal, 1983; Schneider, 1958). Although it has been defined in a variety of ways, it has typically been used to refer to a constellation of traits that include low self-esteem, self-derogation, pessimism, and submissiveness.

The depressive personality, or closely related concepts such as affective personality disorder, was included in most major nosological systems (e.g., DSM-I, DSM-II, ICD-8, ICD-9) prior to DSM-III (American Psychiatric Association, 1980). DSM-III and DSM-III-R (American Psychiatric Association, 1987), however, did not include a specific category for depressive personality. Instead, both documents indicated that the depressive personality was subsumed under the broader rubric of dysthymia.

This assertion has been controversial. Despite the conceptual overlap between dysthymia and depressive personality, there may be important differences between the two constructs. The DSM-III and DSM-III-R criteria for dysthymia emphasize chronic mood disturbance and clinical symptomatology rather than personality traits. Moreover, about half of the dysthymic symptoms included in DSM-III and DSM-III-R are somatic or vegetative, rather than cognitive or affective, in nature (Kocsis & Frances,

1987). Thus, these criteria appear to define a more severe phenotype than is generally implied by the concept of depressive personality (Akiskal, 1989; Goldstein & Anthony, 1988). As a result, a number of investigators have argued that DSM-III and DSM-III-R fail to provide a place for patients with a depressive character structure but whose symptoms are less severe and persistent than those required for a diagnosis of dysthymia (Frances & Cooper, 1981; Goldstein & Anthony, 1988; Gunderson, 1983; Kernberg, 1988).

In light of these concerns, it was proposed (Phillips et al., 1990) that depressive personality be added as a new category in DSM-IV (American Psychiatric Association, 1994), and, eventually, it was included in the DSM-IV appendix. In evaluating the need for such an addition, we must determine whether such a personality can be distinguished from the mood disorders, particularly dysthymia, and whether depressive personality traits are simply the sequelae of prior major depressive episodes (Widiger & Shea, 1991).

This chapter, summarizes the results of two studies, one conducted with an outpatient and the other with a nonclinical sample, which attempted to address these issues. Klein (1990) and Klein and Miller (1993) provide more complete descriptions of the methods and findings of these studies.

Outpatient Study

Methodology

In the first study, 177 subjects were drawn from a larger series of 550 consecutive outpatients at two mental health clinics. Patients were selected on the basis of scores on the General Behavior Inventory (GBI; Depue & Klein, 1988), a screening measure for chronic and recurrent affective symptoms, using a stratified random-sampling method.

Subjects received a structured diagnostic interview based on the Schedule for Affective Disorders and Schizophrenia (SADS; Endicott & Spitzer, 1978) expanded to collect the data necessary to make DSM-III diagnoses and assess borderline and schizotypal personality disorder.

In addition, a series of structured probes was developed to assess Akiskal's (1983) criteria for the depressive temperament. These include seven groups of traits: (1) quiet, introverted, passive, and nonassertive; (2) gloomy, pessimistic, serious, and incapable of fun; (3) self-critical, self-reproaching, and self-derogatory; (4) skeptical, hypercritical, and hard to please; (5) conscientious, responsible, and self-disciplined; (6) brooding and given to worry; and (7) preoccupied with feelings of inadequacy and personal shortcomings. A group of traits was considered present if at least two traits within the group were moderately or highly characteristic of the patient's personality since adolescence or early adulthood and were clearly present outside major depressive episodes. A cutoff of six or more groups of traits was used to define depressive personality.

To assess interrater reliability, a second clinician independently rated audiotapes of 17 interviews. Kappa for a diagnosis of depressive personality was .82.

Patients were also administered the Family History–Research Diagnostic Criteria (FH-RDC; Andreasen et al., 1977) interview to assess psychopathology in all first-degree relatives over age 17. Family history data were age corrected using the Weinberg abridged method (Slater & Cowie, 1971). In order to avoid violating assumptions of independence, probands were used as the unit of analysis by calculating the mean age-corrected rate of disorder within each proband's family.

An attempt was made to conduct blind follow-up assessments for all patients with a DSM-III nonbipolar depression diagnosis 6 months after the initial evaluation. The follow-up included a semistructured interview based on the Longitudinal Interval Follow-up Evaluation (Keller et al., 1987).

Effect of Mood State

To examine the effects of patients' clinical states on the assessment of depressive personality traits, 25 patients who met criteria for a current major depressive episode at the initial evaluation but who reported no more than one or two mild depressive symptoms in the 4 weeks before the follow-up assessment were identified. The mean number of groups of depressive personality traits rated for these subjects in the initial and follow-up evaluations was compared. The difference did not approach significance, indicating that patients' clinical states had minimal effect on the assessment of depressive personality traits.

Association with Mood Disorders

Patients with (n = 53) and without (n = 124) depressive personality were compared on rates of current mood disorders. Subjects with depressive personality exhibited a significantly higher rate of dysthymia (49%) than those without depressive personality (27%) ($\chi^2[1]$ = 7.44, p = .003). Individuals with depressive personality also exhibited a significantly higher rate of primary early onset dysthymia (34%), the subtype that most closely resembles depressive personality, than did those without depressive personality (11%) (χ^2 [1] = 11.40, p < .001). The groups did not differ on rates of bipolar disorders and major depression .

Although dysthymia and depressive personality were significantly associated, the magnitude of the overlap was relatively modest. Only 30% of patients who met one of these sets of criteria met criteria for both. Specifically, 49% of patients with depressive personality met criteria for dysthymia, and 44% of dysthymics met criteria for depressive personality. The concordance between depressive personality and dysthymia, expressed in terms of kappa, was .22. Kappa for the association between depressive personality and primary early onset dysthymia was .26.

Association with Non-Mood Disorders

Patients with and without depressive personality were also compared on rates of lifetime anxiety, eating, and substance use disorders and on borderline and schizotypal personality disorder. A significantly greater proportion of subjects with than without depressive personality met the DSM-III criteria for schizotypal personality (23% vs. 7%) (χ^2[1] = 6.88, p < .01). However, the groups did not differ on any of the other disorders.

Family History

The groups were compared on three family history variables: the proportion of relatives with a history of bipolar disorder, nonbipolar depression, and hospitalization for mood disorders. A significantly higher proportion of relatives of patients with ($\overline{X}$ = .11, SD = .19) than without ($\overline{X}$ = .04, SD = .13) depressive personality had relatives with bipolar conditions (t [170] = 2.52, p = .005). In addition, a significantly higher proportion of subjects with ($\overline{X}$ = .12, SD = .19) than without ($\overline{X}$ = .05, SD = .13) depressive personality had been hospitalized for mood disorders (t [170] = 2.86, p < .005).

Differences between Patients with Dysthymia and Depressive Personality

Finally, we compared patients who met criteria for depressive personality but not dysthymia (n = 27) with those who met criteria for dysthymia but not depressive personality (n = 33) on a selected subset of variables. Patients with dysthymia only obtained significantly higher scores on the GBI depression scale ($\overline{X}$ = 27.0, *SD* = 6.7) than patients with depressive personality only ($\overline{X}$ = 19.5, *SD* = 10.5) (*t* [58] = 3.35, *p* < .001). In addition, dysthymics exhibited significantly higher levels of depression at the 6-month follow-up ($\overline{X}$ = 3.6, *SD* = 1.5) than did subjects with depressive personality only ($\overline{X}$ = 2.5, *SD* = 0.9) (*t* [35] = 2.56, *p* = .007). Subjects with dysthymia only also exhibited a significantly higher rate of nonbipolar depression in relatives ($\overline{X}$ = .40, *SD* = .27) than did subjects with depressive personality only ($\overline{X}$ = .22, *SD* = .25) (*t* [57] = 2.63, *p* = .005). Finally, there was a trend (*p* < .09) for the dysthymics to exhibit a higher rate of borderline personality disorder (42%) than for the patients with depressive personality only (19%) to do so.

Discussion

These data indicate that the depressive personality can be assessed reliably, and that such evaluations are not overly biased by patients' clinical state of depression. The constructs of depressive personality and dysthymia are significantly associated, yet the degree of overlap is modest. Moreover, the two constructs have somewhat different correlates, with dysthymia appearing to be a more symptomatic condition, both cross-sectionally and longitudinally, and showing greater familial aggregation of depression. Depressive personality, on the other hand, may be somewhat more homogeneous, at least with regard to personality style. Finally, despite the modest association between depressive personality and mood disorders in probands, patients with depressive personality had significantly increased rates of mood disorders in relatives compared to subjects without depressive personality. Neither the patients with nor those without depressive personality differed on rates of bipolar disorder and major depression themselves, indicating that depressive personality has a familial relationship to the major mood disorders.

Nonclinical Study

Methodology

One of the limitations of our first study was that the lifetime prevalence of affective disorders was so high in the clinical sample that it was difficult to address the question whether depressive personality traits represented the sequelae of past major depressive episodes. In the second study, we attempted to address this problem and to replicate our previous findings using a college student sample. In order to ensure that there were a sufficient number of cases of depressive personality, as well as a variety of other forms of psychopathology, we selected subjects using a battery of screening inventories designed to identify persons exhibiting features of a number of Axis I and II disorders (Chapman & Chapman, 1985; Depue & Klein, 1988).

One hundred and eighty-five subjects were drawn from a pool of 7,481 Caucasian students taking introductory psychology courses over a 3-year period. Subjects were selected on the basis of their scores on the Physical Anhedonia and Perceptual Aberration Magical Ideation Scales (Chapman & Chapman, 1985) and the GBI (Depue & Klein, 1988) Hypomania and Depression scales. Subjects received the modified version of the SADS described above and the FH-RDC. Again, a cutoff of six of Akiskal's (1983) groups of traits were used to define depressive personality. Interrater reliability, expressed in terms of kappa, was .82 ($n = 54$).

Association with Mood Disorders

Subjects with depressive personality exhibited significantly higher lifetime rates of any mood disorder (61% vs. 18%) (χ^2 [1] = 25.08, $p < .001$), major depression (22% vs. 7%) (χ^2 [1] = 5.41, $p = .02$), and dysthymia (19% vs. 1%) (Fisher's exact test $p = .0002$) than those without depressive personality. In addition, there was a trend ($p < .07$) for a greater proportion of subjects with than without depressive personality to have a lifetime diagnosis of bipolar disorder, bipolar disorder not otherwise specified, or cyclothymia (22% vs. 9%).

Despite the statistical significance of these relationships, the overlap between depressive personality and the mood disorders was modest. The kappas for the associations between depressive personality and any lifetime mood disorder, major depression, and dysthymia were .38, .18, and .25, respectively.

Association with Non-Mood Disorders

The relationships between the depressive personality and the nonaffective disorders were also evaluated, although the prevalence of most of these conditions tended to be low in this sample. Subjects with depressive personality exhibited a marginally significantly ($p = .051$) elevated rate of schizotypal personality disorder (8% vs. 1%). However, subjects with and without depressive personality did not differ significantly on panic disorder, alcohol and drug abuse or dependence, conduct disorder, or borderline personality disorder.

Family History

A significantly greater proportion of first-degree relatives of subjects with ($\overline{X}$ = .29, SD = .36) than without ($\overline{X}$ = .13, SD = .26) depressive personality had a history of affective disorders (t [183] = 2.97, p < .005). In addition, a significantly higher proportion of the relatives of subjects with ($\overline{X}$ = .23, SD = .32) than without ($\overline{X}$ = .12, SD = .26) depressive personality had a history of nonbipolar depression (t [183] = 2.27, p < .02). The two groups did not differ on the proportion of relatives with bipolar disorder, alcoholism, drug abuse, or antisocial personality.

In order to determine whether these differences could be attributed to the higher rate of mood disorders in subjects with depressive personality, the two groups were compared on the rate of affective disorders in relatives after excluding all probands with a lifetime history of mood disorder. Despite the reduced sample size, probands with depressive personality continued to exhibit a significantly higher rate of affective disorders in their first-degree relatives than did probands without depressive personality.

Discussion

Overall, the pattern of findings in the nonclinical study was strikingly similar to that in the outpatient study. In both studies, although depressive personality was significantly associated with dysthymia, the magnitude of the associations was modest. In the nonclinical sample, we were also able to address the question of whether depressive personality traits might represent the sequelae of previous major depressive episodes. Again, although depressive personality was significantly associated with a lifetime diagnosis of major depression, only 22% of subjects with depressive personality had a lifetime history of major depression. Finally, the second study also replicated the earlier finding of an increased rate of mood disorders in the relatives of subjects with depressive personality. Importantly, this was evident even when the analysis was limited to subjects with no personal history of mood disorder.

Conclusion

The results of the two studies, using very different populations, provide convincing evidence that although depressive personality and dysthymia are overlapping constructs, they are not isomorphic, and that the depressive personality is not completely subsumed by existing mood disorders categories. At the same time, although the depressive personality is somewhat distinct from dysthymia and major depression, it appears to have a strong familial relationship to the major affective disorders. These findings suggested the need for revisions in the current nomenclature. Potential options included (1) adding a new category for depressive personality to the DSM-IV, or (2) broadening the criteria for dysthymia to include patients with depressive personality who are not currently eligible for a dysthymia diagnosis. DSM-IV (American Psychiatric Association, 1994) conservatively opted for the first, adding depressive personality to its appendix. This decision highlights the need for further study. Second, our data indicate the importance of assessing depressive personality in family-genetic and high-risk studies of the mood disorders (Akiskal & Akiskal, 1992; Cassano et al., 1992).

Acknowledgments

This work was supported by National Institute of Mental Health Research Grants R01 MH-39628 (to G. A. Miller) and R01 MH-45757 (to D. N. Klein). Joong-Nam Yang, BA, from the University of Illinois at Champaign–Urbana, took part in the research reported in this chapter.

References

Akiskal, H. S. (1983). Dysthymic disorder: Psychopathology of proposed chronic depressive subtypes. *American Journal of Psychiatry, 140,* 11–20.

Akiskal, H. S. (1989). Validating affective personality types. In L. N. Robins & J. E. Barrett (Eds.), *The validity of psychiatric diagnosis* (pp. 217–227). New York: Raven Press.

Akiskal, H. S., & Akiskal, K. (1992). Cyclothymic, hyperthymic and depressive temperaments as subaffective variants of mood disorders. In A. Tasman & M. B. Riba (Eds.), *Annual review* (Vol. 11, pp. 43–62). Washington, DC: American Psychiatric Press.

American Psychiatric Association. (1980). *Diagnostic and statistical manual of mental disorders* (3rd ed.). Washington, DC: Author.

American Psychiatric Association. (1987). *Diagnostic and statistical manual of mental disorders* (3rd ed., rev.). Washington, DC: Author.

American Psychiatric Association. (1994). *Diagnostic and statistical manual of mental disorders* (4th ed.). Washington, DC: Author.

Andreasen, N. C., Endicott, J., Spitzer, R. L., & Winokur, G. (1977). The family history method using diagnostic criteria. *Archives of General Psychiatry, 34,* 1229–1235.

Cassano, G. B., Akiskal, H. S., Perugi, G., Musetti, L., & Savino, M. (1992). The importance of measures of affective temperaments in genetic studies of mood disorders. *Journal of Psychiatric Research, 26,* 257–268.

Chapman, L. J., & Chapman, J. P. (1985). Psychosis proneness. In M. Alpert (Ed.), *Controversies in schizophrenia* (pp. 157–174). New York: Guilford Press.

Depue, R. A., & Klein, D. N. (1988). Identification of unipolar and bipolar affective conditions in clinical and nonclinical populations by the General Behavior Inventory. In D. L. Dunner, E. S. Gershon, & J. E. Barrett (Eds.), *Relatives at risk for mental disorders* (pp. 179–202). New York: Raven Press.

Endicott, J., & Spitzer, R. L. (1978). A diagnostic interview: The Schedule for the Affective Disorders and Schizophrenia. *Archives of General Psychiatry, 35,* 837–844.

Frances, A., & Cooper, A. M. (1981). Descriptive and dynamic psychiatry: A perspective on DSM-III. *American Journal of Psychiatry, 138,* 1198–1202.

Goldstein, W. N., & Anthony, R. N. (1988). The diagnosis of depression and the DSMs. *American Journal of Psychotherapy, 42,* 180–196.

Gunderson, J. (1983). DSM-III diagnoses of personality disorders. In J. P. Frosch (Ed.), *Current perspectives on personality disorders* (pp. 20–39). Washington, DC: American Psychiatric Press.

Keller, M. B., Lavori, P. W., Friedman, B., Nielsen, E., Endicott, J., McDonald-Scott, P., & Andreasen, N. C. (1987). The Longitudinal Interval Follow-up Evaluation: A comprehensive method for assessing outcome in prospective longitudinal studies. *Archives of General Psychiatry, 44,* 540–548.

Kernberg, O. F. (1988). Clinical dimensions of masochism. *Journal of the American Psychoanalytic Association, 36,* 1005–1029.

Klein, D. N. (1990). Depressive personality: Reliability, validity, and relation to dysthymia. *Journal of Abnormal Psychology, 99,* 412–421.

Klein, D. N., & Miller, G. A. (1993). Depressive personality in a nonclinical sample. *American Journal of Psychiatry, 150*(11), 1718–1724.

Kocsis, J. H., & Frances, A. J. (1987). A critical discussion of DSM-III dysthymic disorder. *American Journal of Psychiatry, 144,* 1534–1542.

Phillips, K. A., Gunderson, J. G., Hirschfeld, R. M. A., & Smith, L. E. (1990). A review of the depressive personality. *American Journal of Psychiatry, 147,* 830–837.

Schneider, K. (1958). *Psychopathic personalities.* London: Cassell.

Slater, E., & Cowie, V. (1971). *The genetics of mental disorders.* London: Oxford University Press.

Widiger, T. A., & Shea, T. (1991). Differentiation of Axis I and Axis II disorders. *Journal of Abnormal Psychology, 100,* 399–406.

CHAPTER 8

The Need
for the Concept
of Neurotic Depression
Martin Roth
C. Q. Mountjoy

The majority of patients who present with depression in clinical practice or are identified in epidemiological studies of community samples do not suffer from bipolar, unipolar, psychotic, or endogenous affective disorders. These constitute a relatively small minority of psychiatric disorders in which depression predominates. The majority of cases conform to the picture of a disorder denoted until recently in European psychiatry by the term "neurotic depression."

Some of the misunderstanding in contemporary writing in relation to the large group of disorders of affect that fall outside the boundaries of the bipolar and unipolar disorders (as originally defined) derives from the differences between neurotic depression and the syndromes that have replaced it in European and American psychiatry. In DSM-II (American Psychiatric Association, 1968), neurotic depression was described as a recurrent form of depressive disorder that originated from psychodynamic factors and was also associated with characterological abnormalities of a lasting nature. Specific forms of unconscious conflict were described as responsible for the genesis of the disorder. "Dysthymia" was an attempt by the creators of DSM-III (American Psychiatric Association, 1980) to substitute for this concept a cross-sectional descriptive syndrome that could be submitted to objective investigation and refinement. However, dysthymia has failed, for a number of reasons to be discussed at a later stage, to fill the place in the classification of affective disorders previously occupied by neurotic depression. The abolition of neurotic depression and its assimilation within "major depression" has exerted far-reaching effects upon the classification of affective disorders.

The exclusion of neurotic depression from DSM-III, DSM-III-R (American Psychiatric Association, 1987), and DSM-IV (American Psychiatric Association, 1994), as well as ICD-10 (World Health Organization, 1992) has been justified on the basis of the following criticisms of this disorder as a nosological entity: (1) It lacks a distinctive clinical profile, (2) it cannot be reliably discriminated from other affective and kindred disorders, (3) it lacks diagnostic stability because it emerges on follow-up investigation in the form of a wide range of clinical syndromes that are not within the domain defined by the criteria of neurotic depression, (4) the comorbidity of the disorder with a wide range of other conditions is considered to raise further questions about its clinical identity; and (5) it has no definable pattern of treatment response, and its course and outcome are unpredictable. All these criticisms were fully set out by Bronisch and Klerman (1988).

This chapter compares neurotic depression with dysthymia, which replaced it in DSM-III. We evaluate the criticisms advanced as invalidating neurotic depression and examine whether dysthymia—its substitute—has advanced or muddled the classification of affective disorders in DSM-III and ICD-10. Finally, we argue that the shortcomings of major depressive disorder stem largely from the fact that assimilated within it are two nosologically distinct conditions, "neurotic depression" and "unipolar depression," which cannot be logically accommodated within a single diagnostic entity.

Despite these criticisms, the view that there is a continuum or spectrum of depressive states that extends from bipolar depressions at one extreme to neurotic and kindred depressions at the other continues to be upheld. In a recent authoritative volume devoted to manic–depressive illness, Goodwin and Jamison (1990) cite Kraepelin as having favored a broad spectrum without clear boundaries, which encompassed all forms of depressive and manic–depressive and other affective disorders, including neurotic depression. They quote the following passage from Kraepelin's (1921) treatise on manic–depressive disorder in support of this view: "There is actually an uninterrupted series of transitions to 'periodic melancholia,' at the one end of which those cases stand in which the course is quite indefinite with irregular fluctuations and remissions, while at the other end there are the forms with sharply defined, completely developed morbid picture and definite remissions of long duration" (p. 124).

The body of evidence adduced in recent years favoring a return to Kraepelin's unitary concept of manic disorder is significant and is discussed later. But the broad spectrum of disorders he formulated did not include neurotic depression. Moreover, when discussing the less severe pole of the continuum he was formulating, Kraepelin was almost certainly referring to mild and atypical variants and *formes frustes* of bipolar and unipolar endogenous states. This is supported by the fact that in the eighth edition of his textbook (1913/1986), he described psychogenic depression as one form of "psychopathic disorder," the term used in European psychiatry at the time for the compound group of neurotic states and personality disorders. The reason for his limited attention to psychogenic depression was that Kraepelin spent the greater part of his working life in mental hospitals where neurotic disorders were rare. The huge influx of the commonest forms of depressive disorder into psychiatric practice did not commence until after his death in 1926. Had he survived into this period of daily clinical experience, he might have modified his firmly entrenched opinion that these conditions could not be regarded as forms of illness.

Dysthymia in DSM-III and neurotic depression represent different attempts to delineate the main features of the nonendogenous (and "nonmajor") areas of the affective disorders. The question is whether dysthymia is superior to neurotic depression as a concept for exploring the problems in this area in clinical practice and scientific investigation.

This chapter therefore compares and contrasts neurotic depression and dysthymia in terms of what is known about their clinical profile, biological correlates, long-term course, and discrimination from other disorders. We conclude that there is more evidence for clear differentiation of neurotic depression from other affective disorders and anxiety disorders than for dysthymia. There is more evidence in respect to issues of chronicity, severity, and treatment response to validate neurotic depression than to validate dysthymia. We believe that there is a need for concepts such as neurotic depression to fill the gap left in the classification of affective disorders by its removal. The reinstatement of such a concept would entail some modification of other syndromes in DSM-III and related classifications. In particular, a component of major depression which stems from neurotic depression would have to be eliminated from it. Parallel with this, it would be desirable to reinstate the syndrome of "unipolar depression" as an "endogenous" concept in the descriptive sense as originally conceived by Leonhard (1957).

Because the heterogeneity of neurotic depression is highly influential in having the syndrome declared a "nonentity," we begin with this subject.

The Heterogenity of "Neurotic" Depression

This subject has figured prominently in the arguments to invalidate the concept of neurotic depression as a nosological entity.

Klerman et al. (1979) reviewed the multiple criteria and meanings that have come to be attached to neurotic depression in diagnosis, treatment, and research and in a later paper (Klerman, 1986) called its scientific status into question. In a more recent publication, Bronisch and Klerman (1988) presented the following usages, paraphrased here:

1. Neurotic depression refers to nonpsychotic disorders. It is contrasted with psychotic depression and is a residual category for depressed patients in whom psychotic features are absent.
2. Neurotic depressions are less incapacitating socially than are psychotic depressions. In this sense, the concept refers to a form of depression that caused "mild" impairment of social functioning.
3. The typical picture of neurotic depression lacks endogenous features. This usage defines a nonendogenous form of depression.
4. Neurotic depressions may have a characteristic constellation of symptoms of their own, that is, a distinct profile (Rosenthal & Gudeman, 1967).
5. Neurotic depression follow stressful precipitating events which are usually but not exclusively psychosocial in nature. This usage is synonymous with reactive depression.
6. Neurotic depressions are reactive in another sense than that cited in item 5 in that the level of intensity of symptoms will fluctuate from day to day or hour to hour in response to changes in the environment.
7. Neurotic depressions are the consequence of personality dysfunctions. The episodes of depression represent the latest perturbation of long-standing neurotic personality differentiation and social maladaption. This type of depression is also called characterological depression (Akiskal et al., 1978).
8. Neurotic depressions are the clinical manifestation of underlying unresolved unconscious conflicts. This usage derives from psychoanalytic theory (Nemiah, 1975): (a) mood changes following interpersonal loss, disappointment, or deprivation; (b) a fall in self-esteem; (c) conflicts over the aggressive drive; and (d) a premorbid personality structure comprising narcissism, dependency, and ambivalence.

These eight criteria are presented as distinct and therefore implicitly conflicting and incompatible. Closer evaluation reveals some items to be redundant, others to be untenable in that they conflict with certain lines of evidence, and others still to refer to parochial theories that have not gained general acceptance.

Item 1 is acceptable but redundant. All psychotic depressions are endogenous, and the nonendogenous character of neurotic depressions is already specified in criterion three. Item 4 repeats the essentials of item 3 in other words, and an abbreviated version could be logically assimilated within item 3 because it is neither a separate criterion nor in conflict with others. Item 2 is inessential and invalidated by several lines of evidence, as further discussed in a later section. Neurotic forms of depression are not necessarily less severe than endogenous or even psychotic depression. As far as item 5 is concerned, the early attacks of neurotic depression are usually preceded by stressful life events, and the mood disorder that follows is proportionate and understandable. However, in subsequent attacks stressful precipitating factors may be inconspicuous or absent owing, hypothetically, to the phenomenon of kindling described by Post et al. (1984).

As bipolar and endogenous depressions are also initially precipitated by life events in a proportion of cases, item 5 refers to a nondiscriminating feature that cannot be used as a major criterion for defining it. However, reactivity in the sense described under item 6 is a useful discriminating feature in that unlike the fixed mood of endogenous depressions, that of neurotic depressives generally responds to changes in environment and situation. Item 7 is overstated. Although neurotic depression (as well as dysthymia) commonly occurs in vulnerable personalities, this vulnerability can, in a number of cases, be nonsevere and circumscribed and not the cause of sufficiently severe or lasting maladjustment to warrant a diagnosis of personality disorder.

The psychodynamic factors listed in item 8 have been transposed from DSM-II. They were used mainly in the United States and did not figure in generally accepted definitions or criteria. They were not included among the defining criteria of neurotic depressions in other classification such as ICD-9 or in the many inquiries that attempted to determine their line of demarcation from endogenous and anxiety disorders.

When redundant and inappropriate criteria have been removed from the Bronisch–Klerman list, neurotic depression emerges as a nonendogenous (and nonpsychotic) group of depressions with a distinctive symptoms profile that includes reactivity of mood in changed circumstances, certain vegetative symptoms (described later), and forms of depressive ideation that differ from those that characterize the endogenous states. Neurotic depression occurs in more or less vulnerable personalities, which renders the individual susceptible to varying degrees of breakdown under stress. This clinical profile is delineated in more detail later.

Follow-Up Studies of Neurotic Depression and Dysthymia

The critique of neurotic depression derived from "multiple meanings" signifying a heterogeneous entity has been reinforced by the results of a number of follow-up studies (Akiskal et al., 1978; Bronisch et al., 1985). Neurotic depression showed diagnostic instability when observed in the course of long-term follow-up studies. The wide range of diagnoses that evolved was construed as signifying that it comprised a heterogeneous blend of different disorders. The findings were influential among others in the decisions to exclude neurotic depression from DSM-III-R and to substitute dysthymia.

Akiskal et al. (1978) in an important study in relation to this controversy, followed up 100 outpatients with "mild depressive states" described as reactive or neurotic. After 3 to 4 years, 38 of the 100 patients had developed a "nonaffective" disorder, 18 patients were rediagnosed as bipolar disorder, and 22 as unipolar depressive illness. Ten patients were judged to suffer from a depressive disorder "secondary to medical–surgical illness" and 12 patients from "undiagnosed or probable" depression. Other conditions identified were diagnosed as nonaffective anxiety and phobic neuroses, obsessive–compulsive states (4), Briquet's disorder (8), alcoholism (7), antisocial personality (27), and schizophrenia or schizoaffective disorder (3). The index diagnoses were based on the DSM-II criteria for neurotic depression and Washington University criteria for depression. All available case records were reviewed and family members interviewed. In the light of this, it is perhaps surprising that although there was family history of affective illness, 20 of the patients during prospective observation were diagnosed as suffering from bipolar or unipolar illness, and 10 of these 40 patients developed hypomanic episodes while receiving antidepressant treatment in the follow-up period. None of these patients was correctly diagnosed at index admission and excluded on the basis of the family history. Those with such history should have been disqualified.

Turning to nonaffective disorders, alcoholic dependence may develop as a complication of neurotic depression as well as other emotional disorders. The alcoholism diagnosed in seven cases cannot be construed as refuting or being inconsistent with the index diagnosis of neurotic depression made at the commencement of the study. No less than 22 of the patients with a nonaffective disorder exhibited neurotic symptoms.

As these features may have reflected a coloring added by the background personality, it is not clear why they were judged inconsistent with the index diagnosis of neurotic depression, which may have gone into a phase of remission. The concept of secondary depression arising in association with medical–surgical illness is open to criticism. Somatic illness may be a precipitant; the strength of its association with depression is difficult to determine. Many such patients in a remission following antidepressant treatment will respond even in a chronic somatic disorder such as old age. In other cases, physical illness recovers but depression continues.

The findings and conclusions of Akiskal et al. (1978, 1979) and Bronisch et al. (1985) are at variance with those of the follow-up studies of anxiety and depressive disorders done two decades ago (Kerr et al., 1972). Standardized comprehensive diagnostic interviews were undertaken throughout the 3- to 4-year period of the study at 6-month intervals. There was very little change or crossover over time between the four index diagnoses: neurotic depression, endogenous or psychotic depression, agoraphobia, or general anxiety disorder. The outcome of those with depressive disorders was more favorable in respect of clinical status and social adaptation to that of patients with anxiety disorder (Kerr et al., 1972; Schapira et al., 1972).

An Australian follow-up study has adduced additional evidence regarding the distinction between endogenous and neurotic depressions. Andrews et al. (1990) reported that whereas personality features in endogenous depressions accounted for only 2% of variance in respect of the outcome recorded in their long-term study in the case of neurotic depressions, 20% of the variance was explained by personality variables. It seems unlikely that a group of conditions as heterogeneous as those that emerged from the comprehensive studies of Akiskal et al. (1978, 1979; Akiskal, 1990) could have yielded a result of this nature. The most likely explanation of the disparity is that criteria used by European and related investigators define a different clinical profile from that identified by DSM-III and other criteria.

It has been tacitly assumed that dysthymia possessed stability as a clinical syndrome presumably because a chronic course was one of the principal diagnostic criteria that defined it. This assumption has been rebutted by a number of recent inquiries. Sieveright and Tyrer (1990) compared the features and outcome of 48 patients with dysthymia and those of 61 patients with panic disorder and 50 with general anxiety disorder over a 12-month period. Ten of the 48 dysthymic patients required admission to hospital despite the fact that inpatient treatment was reserved in this particular facility for those with serious conditions. This finding was inconsistent with the view that patients diagnosed as dysthymic all suffered from "mild" disorder. Only a quarter of those with an initial diagnosis of dysthymic condition continued to satisfy criteria for this disorder 4 months later. The remainder were given diagnoses such as major depressive episode, panic disorder, melancholia, agoraphobia, and no psychiatric disorder (21%). A diagnosis of personality disorder was elicited in 50% of patients. Higher rates were found by Roy et al. (1985).

Roy et al. (1985) reached the same conclusion as Akiskal regarding dysthymia from observations of patients with neurotic depression. They questioned the validity of dysthymia as a nosological entity. There is nothing to choose between neurotic depression and dysthymia in this respect. The relatively large overlap between dysthymia and anxiety disorders reported by Roy et al., among others, has further implications, which are discussed in the next section.

Diagnosis of Nonendogenous and Nonmajor Depressions

It was understandable that the architects of DSM-III would pay special attention to the definition of those forms of mood disorder that are distinct from bipolar and unipolar forms of manic–depressive illness. These represent by far the most highly prevalent forms of affective disorder encountered in all forms of clinical practice and epidemiological studies of community samples. Thus the definition of these disorders must be reliable, valid, and as sharply discriminative from other disorders as existing knowledge permits.

The main criteria of dysthymia are as follows:

1. A mild or moderate depressive syndrome that pursues a chronic course with a duration of 2 years or longer, which must not be the residual aftermath of major depression. During a 2-year period the main symptoms should never have been absent for longer than 2 months at a time.
2. A presenting clinical profile comprising two of six symptoms, five of which are among the less specifically diagnostic features of major depression. The symptoms are disturbance of appetite, insomnia or hypersomnia, low energy, low self-esteem, poor concentration, and feelings of hopelessness.
3. Early (before 21 years) or late (at age 21 or later) onset.
4. An associated personality disturbance, which may warrant a diagnosis of personality disorder along Axis II.
5. Major depression in the first 2 years. Mania or hypomania at any time, schizophrenia or delusional disorder, or contributions by an organic factor are exclusion criteria.

Comparison of Characteristics

We now consider these clinical features of dysthymia in more detail and compare them with those that characterize neurotic depression.

Dysthymia is described as a mild or moderate version of major depression with fewer symptoms and a chronic course. However, difference in severity of symptoms provides a weak basis for the differentiation of any hypothetical syndrome from other syndromes. In the case of a psychiatric disorder that is subject to recurrence, the symptoms of the attacks that follow index examination and diagnosis may prove of greater or lesser severity. In the case of relapse into a more severe illness, a second diagnosis has to be added to the less severe disorder diagnosed at the index stage, where severity has been a major criterion for separating the syndromes from each other. This generates confusion. Each of these ostensibly separate conditions, in this case dysthymia and major depression, draws on the same range of clinical features in its presenting phenomenology. The allocation of different names to what is mainly a variation in severity conceals the true relationship between the phenomena. This describes the situation that pertains to dysthymia. Low-grade symptomatology is described as dysthymic. When an intensification of symptoms occurs in the low-grade chronic disorder, the diagnosis is major depressive episode ostensibly superimposed upon a disorder relatively distinct from it, namely, dysthymia.

In contrast, the description of neurotic depression does not include statements about severity. Variation in severity in the manifestation of recurrent illnesses over a period is a common finding in psychiatric disorders. It is the clinical profile and not severity of illness of neurotic depressions that differentiates it from endogenous unipolar and bipolar disorders. Although the endogenous disorders tend *in the main* to be more severe, pervasive, and disabling, each of these two main groups varies in severity. Consequently, a number of patients with neurotic depression suffer from attacks of illness more severe and disabling than the depressive attacks of some bipolar and unipolar cases. On the other hand, endogenous depression may be relatively "silent" and inconspicuous and therefore liable to escape notice. It is also liable, on the basis of the distinctions in terms of severity between "major" and "minor" depression in DSM-III, to be described as dysthymia. This error in diagnosis may prove particularly inappropriate in old age when nonsevere depressions with few symptoms have been shown to carry serious suicidal risk (Barraclough et al., 1974).

Neurotic depression is, in the majority of cases, an episodic disorder in which attacks are separated by relatively clear intermissions broken by no more than mild occasional symptoms. It is only after years of illness, commonly in old age, that the aftermath of despondency that follows attacks of illness becomes sufficiently pronounced and confluent to acquire the features of a chronic disorder. However, many patients with neurotic depression recover from their attacks with appropriate treatment and may function well for years despite repeated episodes of illness requiring treatment. Moreover, work and social and familial relationships may be well sustained over long periods.

The Chronicity of Dysthymia

There is no formal evidence that chronicity is a consistent characteristic of all nonendogenous depressions. The chronicity criterion is a disadvantage of leaving no room in the classification of affective disorders for recurrent forms that have in the past been recognized as one variety of neurotic illness. These conditions, particularly when they are severe, are liable to receive a diagnosis of major depression. But this condition is also the repository of what used to be described as unipolar depression. This is unfortunate, because, as we argue later, unipolar depression belongs indubitably with bipolar depression as a closely related form of manic–depressive disorder. Major depressive disorder constitutes a mixture of different forms of disturbance of affect with consequences for the remainder of the classification of affective disorders that we consider here.

The place of neurotic depression as conceived in the past is now occupied in ICD-10 by a "recurrent depressive disorder." This syndrome may be mild or moderate. There is also a severe form of this syndrome which may present without psychotic symptoms or as a separate category with psychotic symptoms. The nonpsychotic forms of this syndrome were clearly intended to be substituted for neurotic depression because psychogenic depression and reactive depression are explicitly described as being subsumed under the rubric of recurrent depressive disorder. (In DSM-III and DSM-IV, dysthymia is also described in parentheses as depressive neurosis.) The episode is said to last between 3 and 12 months with a median duration of about 6 months, recurrence being less common than in bipolar disorder. Recovery is usually complete between episodes—"but a minority of patients may develop a persistent depression mainly in old age."

In seeking to exclude neurotic depression as far as possible, this classification runs into the same difficulties as those manifest in DSM-IV. Although the affinities with neurotic depression are declared, it is stipulated that recurrent depressive disorder should be the diagnosis even if there are brief episodes of elevation of mood and overactivity, which fulfill the criteria of hypomania. These conditions would, in light of the recent literature, be classed by many clinicians and investigators as bipolar (Cassano et al., 1992). Unipolar disorders, which do not figure in ICD-10, will also have been incorporated. ICD-10 makes clear, however, that there is a condition such as neurotic depression in which recurrent attacks of mood disorder occur lasting on an average of about 6 months separated by periods of clear remission. This is, however, assimilated within a syndrome akin to Kraepelin's manic–depressive illness.

Life Events in Neurotic Depression and Dysthymia

Neurotic depression frequently (but not always) evolves following some traumatic situation such as a bereavement or loss, demotion, or failure. This mode of onset characterizes first attacks in particular. A stressful event preceded illness in the great majority of the 2,000 soldiers studied by Slater (1943) during World War II. The severity of the threat or trauma provided an approximate measure of the vulnerability of the personality and its predisposition to breakdown. Trivial circumstances sufficed to precipitate neurotic disorder in poorly endowed, immature, and emotionally labile persons. But it took an overwhelming type of trauma to precipitate a neurotic depression (or other neurotic illness) in emotionally strong, vigorous, well-integrated individuals with a record of past achievement. Inferences drawn from severity of precipitating stress were on the whole corroborated by systematic investigation of the previous history, achievement, and personality traits of the individuals concerned. Generalizations cannot be validly made from circumstances in which a substantial proportion of the persons involved were exposed to the danger of annihilation in battle. But the findings provide a rough guide for evaluation in ordinary civilian life.

According to the account provided in DSM-III, dysthymia implicitly differs from neurotic depressions in this respect in that the condition is stated to commence insidiously ("without clear onset") and in the absence of any relevant trauma in childhood or adolescence. However, as a high proportion of patients present first in middle life or old age, the circumstances in which the first or early attacks occurred may have been obscured by the experiences during the period that has intervened.

The view that the onset of dysthymia differs from that of neurotic depression—being insidious and without antecedent life events—has been called into question by the findings of Sieveright and Tyrer (1990), who conducted an inquiry into 48 patients with dysthymia (diagnosed by the DSM-III criteria) who were compared with groups of patients with general anxiety disorder and panic disorder. Of 48 of the dysthymic patients, 42 suffered from onerous life events in impressive association with the onset of their illness; in 33 of these patients, the events were related to illness or death in associates or relatives or stresses in connection with marriage, children, or sexual relationships. In all three groups the number of life events experienced by patients was just under three incidents. The degree of stress was assessed by calculating the consensus-derived scores with the degree of stressful intensity. There was no significant difference in respect to the number of stresses between the three groups as estimated by these techniques (Tyrer, 1989).

Neurotic depression was recognized in traditional European psychiatry arising in a "constitutional" or personality setting which played a significant part in the genesis of the disorder. In the textbook *Clinical Psychiatry* (Slater & Roth, 1977, p. 78), personality background was described as follows: "The past personality of the patient shows a greater lability than usual. He is elated by pleasant occurrences, cast down by disappointments—likely to brood upon unpleasant events, to be unable to throw things off easily and even constantly of a mildly pessimistic nature." Hirschfeld (1990) recorded similar findings in a study of a large group of patients with affective disorder including dysthymia. He stated: "They have extremely low levels of emotional strength and are likely to break down under stress. They are likely to be moody and fearful. They are very introverted and shy, avoiding social interactions" (p. 76).

Comorbidity

Bronisch et al. (1985) reported a high degree of comorbidity of neurotic depression with other disorders in their Munich follow-up study. This is cited by Bronisch and Klerman (1988) among the lines of evidence that impugn the nosological validity of neurotic depression. However, were comorbidity with other disorders permitted to invalidate nosological entities, all the disorders classed under the heading of neurosis would be eliminated, including panic–agoraphobic disorder, obsessive–compulsive states, social phobia, somatoform disorders, and anorexia nervosa (Roth 1977, 1984). This criticism ignores the criterion of clinical salience of one cluster of features to which diagnostic terms used for the neuroses refer. This cluster survives in these disorders as in neurotic depression, whereas the coloring of other features varies and often goes into abeyance. Nor does this criticism take into account the much greater instability, in a long-term perspective, of pathoplastic features, which lend a variable coloring to the clinical picture. These features stem from the basic personality and from other reactive and secondary features which are not consistently manifest from one episode of illness to the next.

Akiskal et al. (1978) and Bronisch et al. (1985) did not quote the only investigation in which patients with neurotic depression among other disorders were examined in a follow-up by independent investigators ignorant of the initial index diagnosis made on the basis of strict diagnostic criteria. This inquiry reported a high degree of stability for all four groups of affective and anxiety disorders investigated, including neurotic depression (Kerr et al., 1972; Schapira et al., 1972).

Heredity

Inconsistent results from investigations of the heredity of neurotic depression have also been cited as calling into question the validity of neurotic depression as a nosological entity. This claim of inconsistency is not supported by the genetic evidence on record, including the studies cited by Bronisch and Klerman themselves. Two authoritative twin studies (Slater & Shields, 1969; Torgersen, 1983) were unable to bring to light any evidence for a hereditary basis for nonpsychotic or neurotic depression. In neurotic depressives' families, risk of first-degree relatives for affective disorder did not differ from the risk in the general population. However, the presence or absence of precipitants contributes little to the discrimination of neurotic from endogenous depression (Carney et al., 1965); endogenous depressions are also triggered in many cases by adverse life events, although the affective disturbance that follows is disproportionate in its severity and duration.

In contrast, a large body of evidence comprehensively reviewed in the recent text of Goodwin and Jamison (1990) established a significant genetic contribution to the causation of bipolar and unipolar depressions. Major depression as defined in DSM-III proves also to be a familial disorder (Goldin & Gershon, 1986). But the findings may arise from the fact that unipolar depression is one among other components of major depression. Neurotic depression is the largest other constituent of the syndrome. Falide et al. (1987) reported similar results to those of Torgersen (1986).

The other imputation, that the absence of any definite hereditary basis invalidates neurotic depression as a psychiatric syndrome, would also eliminate anorexia nervosa, some forms of somatoform disorder, and the dissociative and conversion forms of hysteria as demonstrated by the classical twin studies of Slater (1953). When a specific genetic basis can be demonstrated for a hypothetical psychiatric disorder, it contributes substantially to its establishment as a distinct clinical and biological entity. But the absence of evidence for a hereditary basis cannot be logically employed to impugn its validity. This negative finding separates neurotic depression from unipolar depression in the causation of which there is a well-established hereditary component. This disorder now forms the greater part of major depressive illness as defined in DSM-III. Neurotic depression is also differentiated from dysthymia by virtue of the boundary line defined between it and anxiety disorders (as described earlier). But Sieveright and Tyrer (1990) found dysthymia to be indistinguishable from anxiety disorders on a range of variables. These results call into question the validity of describing dysthymia as synonymous with depressive neurosis both in DSM-IV and in ICD-10.

Personality Setting

The differentiation of depressive disorders from anxiety states presents considerable difficulty in many cases, and some workers deny the existence of a clear line of demarcation between them. The evidence that has emerged from inquiries into the problem of discrimination in this area has a significant bearing on the "neurotic" form of "nonendogenous" depressions.

In the first Newcastle inquiry into the relationship between depressive and anxiety disorders, evidence from phenomenology, treatment response, outcome, and character of the predictive indices developed from multivariate statistical analyses supported the binary nature of the anxiety and depressive disorders (Roth et al., 1972; Kerr et al., 1972; Schapira et al., 1972; Kerr et al., 1974). Principal components analysis followed by a discriminant function analysis showed the great majority of those with anxiety disorder to be located in one mode of a bimodal distribution and most depressions in the other (Gurney et al., 1972) with little overlap.

In a subsequent inquiry (Mountjoy & Roth, 1982a, 1982b), patients with endogenous depression were therefore omitted because they might have made a disproportionate contribution to the separations achieved. As the depressed patients were neurotic depressives *alone*, the results are more closely relevant for this chapter. Information concerning premorbid personality and the developmental history and early behavioral patterns of patients was recorded with the aid of a large number of carefully defined items at the time of interview but was not used in the first stage of the study. The published findings were derived from analysis of the presenting clinical features alone (Mountjoy & Roth, 1982a, 1982b). The multivariate statistical analysis had at this stage again yielded separation of anxiety and depressive disorders in respect to both clinical profile and the distribution of discriminant coefficients derived from scores on nine rating scales for anxiety and depression that were administered to all patients.

The data relating to the personality and developmental items that had been defined and recorded in the original Newcastle study (but not included in the inquiry of 1982) were analyzed (Roth & Mountjoy, 1992, and unpublished observations). As the number of variables exceeded the number of cases, the items were reduced from 65 to 37 by eliminating those elicited with a frequency of more than 90% or less than 10%. The remaining variables were further reduced by carrying out three separate discriminant function analyses and selecting the best discriminators from each.

The discriminant function analysis was carried out using the Mahalanobis technique to maximize the distance between groups. Definite cases were defined as those in which the clinical diagnosis made on the basis of predefined criteria proved congruent with that made on the basis of the Newcastle Anxiety–Depressive Diagnostic Scale (Gurney et al., 1972). In a minority of patients these two separate assessments yielded contradictory diagnoses. These patients were classed as "doubtful" and omitted from the initial stage of the analysis.

A highly significant separation (p < .0004) was achieved between the depressive group on the one hand and the combined anxiety and phobic group combined on the other. In the analysis of the patients of both sexes, 78% of grouped cases were correctly classified into one or the other of the groups in which a definite diagnosis had proved possible. The doubtful cases were also allotted in most cases to one or other of the two modes of the distribution. The separation of grouped cases (78% correct) was highly significant statistically (p < .0004).

But there were clear differences in the profiles of the two sexes. In the analysis of the males, items that carried significant discriminating weights included anticipatory anxiety, evanescent enthusiasms, premorbid somatic anxiety, and easily upset. All these items allocated patients to the anxiety part of the distribution. Those with discriminating weights in the opposite direction classified the patients into the depressive part of the distribution and included exploitation of other emotions and a low score for neuroticism on the MPI (Maudsley Personality Inventory; Eysenck, 1959). In the male group, none of the childhood neurotic traits had a significant discriminative power. The proportion of patients correctly classified totaled 74%. These separations did not quite reach statistical significance (p = .085).

A different picture emerged in women. The most highly discriminating feature was evanescent enthusiasms, followed in order of importance by childhood bedwetting, childhood nail biting, and MPI neuroticism score, all of which correlated with a diagnosis of anxiety. The weighting of premorbid somatic anxiety was not significant statistically. The significant features that allocated patients to the depressive part of distribution were childhood temper tantrums and impulsive behavior. Of grouped female cases, 87% were correctly classified, and the correlation proved highly significant statistically (p = .0000).

There are two points to be made about this inquiry. The first relates to the finding that was possible to separate patients with anxiety disorders from those with depression employing only simple personality tests and a number of predefined descriptive clinical items of overt behavior and adjustment. In the earlier inquiries into the clinical features of anxiety and depressive disorders, clear lines of demarcation were achieved between the two main groups but also between neurotic depression alone and anxiety disorders (Mountjoy & Roth, 1982a, 1982b). In this last inquiry, neurotic depression alone was also shown to be distinct from general anxiety disorders, agoraphobic and other phobic states having been excluded from one of the analyses.

The absence of any definable personality characteristics was among the criticisms leveled by Bronisch and Klerman (1988) against the status of neurotic depression as a valid syndrome. They cited the findings reported in the study by von Zerssen (1982) in support of this view. However, on the strength of this criterion von Zerssen's observations would invalidate virtually every syndrome in psychiatry with the exception of melancholia. None of the other psychiatric disorders studied by him with the aid of the scales of Tellenbach (1976) were found to have a distinctive personality setting.

It has therefore proved possible to draw a relatively sharp line of demarcation between depressive disorders and anxiety states even when endogenous depressions are excluded from the depressive states. It has been possible to achieve discrimination in the most problematic boundary of the affective disorders: that which separates the nonendogenous or neurotic depressions from anxiety states. This line of separation was achieved in the analysis of data both derived from structured clinical interviews and obtained with the aid of rating scales for anxiety and depression in the same group of patients and with measures of premorbid personality (Mountjoy & Roth, 1982a, 1982b; Roth & Mountjoy, 1982, 1992).

There was a clear difference in the last study between men and women in respect to the profile of premorbid personality and early behavioral patterns of those with anxiety and depressive disorders. The clinical, personality, and biological measurements for patients with anxiety and depressive disorders should therefore be analyzed separately as well as jointly for the two sexes, because significant findings for women may be diluted and therefore obscured by negative findings for men, and vice versa.

The discrimination between the anxiety and depressive groups of disorders has surfaced again in relation to the DSM-III classification and its successors. It is the difficulty encountered in attempting to differentiate dysthymia from general anxiety disorder (Riskind et al., 1987) that is of particular relevance in the present context. In this respect, and in relation to other characteristics described in this chapter, nonendogenous or neurotic depression has a more sharply defined clinical profile than dysthymia, which has replaced neurotic depression in DSM-III and its successors.

Independence of Endogenous and Neurotic Depressions

The validity of the concept of neurotic depression depends on the clarity with which it can be differentiated from the endogenous group of affective disorders. This applies equally to the concept of dysthymia. In fact, if the evidence for the binary nature of the psychotic forms of depression on the one hand and the neurotic forms on the other is discounted, the classification of affective illness loses order and cohesion (Roth, 1979; Roth & Barnes, 1981).

The independence of these two main groups of affective disorder has been a subject of controversy for a long time, and only a brief review is attempted here. These groups have been discriminated from each other by a number of factor analytic and discriminant function analyses (Kiloh & Garside, 1963; Rosenthal & Klerman, 1966; Garside et al., 1971; Kiloh et al., 1972; Raskin & Crook, 1976). Mendels and Cochrane (1968), reviewing seven factor analytic studies, concluded that the consensus of evidence was in support of the independence of the endogenous and neurotic disorders. Comprehensive studies of affective, anxiety, and kindred disorders that embody these and other findings have been published (Roth, 1978, 1979; Roth & Barnes, 1981).

The clinical picture of endogenous depression is made up of a characteristic cluster of symptoms described in similar terms in all the widely accepted international classifications of affective disorder. The disorder has a typically recurrent course with episodes separated by remissions, and it shows a significantly better response to the main groups of antidepressant drugs and electroconvulsive treatment than do nonendogenous disorders (Ball & Kiloh, 1959; Kiloh & Ball, 1961; Kiloh et al., 1962; Kiloh & Garside, 1963; Carney et al., 1965; Hickie et al., 1990). The clinical profile that emerges from investigations of the diagnosis of neurotic depression and its discrimination from other disorders is described later.

Clear separation in the form of bimodal distributions has not been found by some investigators (Kendell, 1968; Kendell & Gourlay, 1970; Ni Bhrolchain et al., 1979), although the unimodality of some published distributions is dubious. However, continuous distributions do not invalidate bimodal distributions, which have repeatedly emerged from different investigations. It is well-known that two or more modes may be concealed under a continuous distribution, particularly when relatively small numbers of cases or unrepresentative samples have been analyzed. A number of cluster analytic studies have also confirmed the clear categorical status of endogenous forms of disorder (Pilowsky et al., 1969; Paykel, 1971, 1972; Matussek et al., 1982).

Some workers have interpreted their findings as more consistent with a continuum of depressive disorders ranging from endogenous and related forms at one extreme and the neurotic depressions at the other (Kendell, 1968). But none of the distributions published could be described as unequivocally unimodal. The interpretations made of such ostensibly continuous distributions are also controversial. The view that such curves represent variations of severity of depression is inconsistent with several lines of evidence. Endogenous and psychotic depressions are not merely more severe forms of nonendogenous depressions. Such interpretations are inconsistent with the better prognosis and superior treatment response with the whole range of biological treatments, including pharmacological and electroconvulsive therapy in patients with endogenous depression. Only a qualitative distinction, a difference in kind between endogenous and nonendogenous (bipolar and unipolar) depressions, can be viewed as consistent with such findings.

Neurotic depressions are not necessarily less severe than endogenous conditions. Affective disturbance may be more intense and florid, and considerable suicidal risk is present in a substantial proportion of cases. In contrast, endogenous states may be nonsevere and unobtrusive, particularly in late middle age and old age. It is the "silence" of the depressions of later life that conceals the suicidal risk among many elderly who carry out carefully planned suicide.

A number of recent investigations provided strong support for categorical definition and independence of endogenous depression. Parker et al. (1990) in Sydney isolated a cluster of features subsumed under "retardation." Retardation has long been stressed as a central feature of melancholia and its subgroups of psychotic and endogenous depression (Rosenthal & Gudeman, 1967; Kay et al., 1969). Using multivariate analyses, Parker et al. defined a "core" group of 15 signs that differentiated psychotic/endogenous and nonendogenous depressives in two separate samples. This core cluster proved to be highly correlated with clinical DSM-III and Research Diagnostic Criteria (Spitzer et al., 1978) diagnoses of melancholia, suggesting that the endogenous group could be defined with the aid of objective phenomenological features. Similar observations favoring the discriminating power of psychomotor retardation have been recorded by a French group of observers (Widlocher, 1987).

A separate investigation of electroconvulsive therapy response in 35 patients by the Sydney groups (Hickie et al., 1990) demonstrated that psychomotor disturbance as assessed by the core rating system successfully predicted the response to electroconvulsive treatment in patients with a retarded form of melancholia. As delusions and hallucinations were ineffective predictors in contrast to retardation, these findings supported the kinship and continuity of the endogenous, melancholic, and psychotic forms of depression.

Another Australian investigation, which determined long-term outcome of endogenous and neurotic depression (Andrews et al., 1990), demonstrated that whereas in endogenous depression personality factors accounted for only 2% of the variance in outcome, in neurotic depression they accounted for 20% of the variance. Personality measures in isolation provide only a small proportion of the body of evidence that defines the premorbid status of these patients. The addition of developmental findings; record of occupational, sexual, and interpersonal adjustment; and evidence regarding achievements and failures which are regularly elicited in the course of comprehensive psychiatric examination might reveal in the judgment of these authors an even larger contribution by indices of premorbid characteristics to variance in respect to treatment in the neurotic depressions in particular.

Some Special Syndromes of Neurotic Depression

In the large and poorly mapped area of affective disorders that are outside the bounds of the endogenous depressions, both bipolar and unipolar, the last few decades have seen a proliferation of syndromes that do not differ significantly from neurotic depression in respect to the presenting features of the mental state. A number of these conditions have been endowed with a special status through the application of some adjectival prefix derived from the personality setting which has endowed the present clinical syndrome with a distinctive coloring.

The syndrome of hostile depression has been identified by a number of authors (Overall et al., 1966; Lorr et al., 1973; Paykel, 1971). Kiloh et al. (1972) and Paykel et al. (1971), in particular, in each case in large patient samples, make it clear that the disorder is related to the neurotic forms of depression. The "hostile" group has some of the characteristics of the histrionic–aggressive patients of Lazare and Klerman (1968), the "angry depressives" of Grinker et al. (1961) and the "self-pitying constellation" of Rosenthal and Gudeman (1967), and the "chronic characterological syndrome" of Schildkraut (1970). Klein and Davis (1969) described the concept of "hysteroid dysphoria." This bears some resemblance to the hostile group of depressions, but the personality features have been delineated in more detail in this case. These individuals are described as oversensitive, overdependent on applause, and liable to eat and sleep to excess, to become fatigued easily, and to exhibit a shallow labile mood in the course of their illness.

In no case has the personality profile of these groups of patients been studied with the aid of systematic structured clinical evaluation and standardized measures of personality. DSM-IV has paid no attention to these disorders. However, as they continue to figure in the literature, it would be desirable to determine their precise status. The extent to which they can be accommodated within the concept of dysthymia is unknown at the present time.

Further observations are needed to determine where these syndromes belong in the classification of affective disorders. If they are all variants of nonendogenous depression that have been accorded separate nosological status on account of epiphenomenal features emanating from the personality setting, they should preferably be classed as neurotic depression, and accorded a personality diagnosis derived from clinical examination and/or Axis II of DSM-IV. Entities should not be multiplied unnecessarily, and it would be undesirable for this plethora of nonendogenous forms of depression to overcrowd and obscure the already complex literature of this group of disorders.

Systematic studies should be undertaken to determine whether these hostile self-pitying hysteroid dysphoric depressions refer by different names to one and the same clinical syndrome. The personality or other features that separate them from the main nonendogenous categories of neurotic depression and dysthymia remain to be identified.

Delineating Neurotic Depression

Bronisch and Klerman (1988) state that neurotic depression is deficient in its phenomenological discrimination from other disorders. This statement is at variance with the greater part of the literature that deals with this subject. Other inquiries that defined a line of separation between neurotic depression and anxiety disorders with limited overlap have also been summarized. We have finally separated neurotic depression from unipolar illness. Table 8.1 summarizes what we consider the distinctive features of neurotic depression.

Bronisch and Klerman (1988) hold that neurotic depression has no persistent or unitary clinical features. But the description they have compiled from the studies of Matussek et al. (1982), Winokur (1985), and Zimmerman et al. (1987), and the results of the Newcastle–

TABLE 8.1. Clinical Features of "Neurotic Depression"

Leading symptoms of presenting illness

Depression of mood more intense and disabling than normal sadness but lacking "distinct" quality described by "endogenous" cases.

Mood appropriately reactive to adverse or favorable changes in life circumstances and to everyday events.

Somatic complaints with hypochondriacal concern.

Initial insomnia or interrupted sleep. Either no diurnal variation or worsening of symptoms in evening.

Prominent but variable anxiety.

Hostility, irritability, and anger (exaggeration of premorbid traits) in a proportion but not all cases.

Self-pity and/or tendency to blame others. Absence of self-reproach or guilt.

Demanding, manipulative, self-dramatizing behavior in those with hysterical premorbid traits.

Absence of psychomotor retardation.

Personality

There is evidence of maladjustment and vulnerability in the premorbid personality which may color the symptomatology of illness. It does not necessarily cause continual or serious disability in personal and social roles. It is not incompatible with high achievement. Although there is personal maladjustment and disability in a proportion of cases, diagnosis of personalilty disorder is not always justified.

Life events

Life events impressively and understandably related to onset of symptoms in a high proportion of cases

History of illness longer than in endogenous cases.

Onset

Symptoms commence some months before contact in association with stress.

Course

Course is usually episodic with clear remission.

The duration of attacks varies in accordance with personality assets and life situation.

Family history

A history of affective disorder in first-degree relatives is usually lacking. Some relatives described as "nervous" or "emotional" without record of illness.

A positive family history does not by itself invalidate clinical diagnosis.

Treatment response

A proportion of patients respond to treatment with cognitive therapy (Beck, 1967), interpersonal psychotherapy (Klerman et al., 1984), pharmacotherapy (Ball & Kiloh, 1959), electroconvulsive therapy (Carney et al., 1965), or a combination of these methods. Recurrence is frequent, but chronicity is a feature only in those with severe personality difficulties or disorder and after many years of illness.

Cambridge inquiries (Roth et al., 1972; Mountjoy & Roth, 1982a, 1982b; Roth & Mountjoy, 1992) make the negative statements untenable. Actually, Table 8.1 incorporates many features that Bronisch and Klerman cited as being nonspecific. However, their own descriptive outline with some added features from the literature refutes their assertion that the syndrome of neurotic depression lacks a clear clinical identity. Many of the added and modified items have been drawn from studies in which multivariate statistical methods were used to estimate the diagnostic discriminating and predictive value of groups of patients with depressive illness. The profile that emerges is as well rooted in clinical observation, long-term follow-up studies, and the results of therapeutic trials as is that of major depression.

Normal sadness is among the features cited by Bronisch and Klerman. It is perhaps more precise to state that the depression of neurotic depressives is of greater intensity and more disabling than normal sadness, although, unlike endogenous depression, sufferers do not describe it as "distinct" in quality. Other features such as self-pity, multiple somatic complaints, and reactivity to the outside world have emerged consistently from multivariate analyses of cohorts of patients as belonging to the constellation of neurotic depressive features. As far as multiple nonserious suicide attempts are concerned, only a small number of neurotic depressives make suicidal attempts and not all are nonserious. Some severe cases deliberately choose lethal methods. Others die unintentionally following impulsive attempts using the most accessible means, which may be a bottle full of tricyclic antidepressants.

The features in Table 8.1 are listed as irritability, hostility, blaming others, a tendency to complain, and demanding behavior. This describes the profile well, but only in a limited proportion of cases is a diagnosis of personality disorder justified. In many patients, probably the majority in a representative sample, the condition is episodic, and the periods that intervene are marked only by short-lived emotional disturbance that does not require admission to hospital or cessation of work. Such patients may be vulnerable to certain types of stress and maladjusted to circumscribed ways without meeting criteria for a diagnosis of personality disorder.

"Life events" listed as a "pathogenetic factor" needs qualification. In one of the larger inquiries into endogenous and neurotic depression, "no precipitants" had a relatively low loading as compared with other features on a statistically derived endogenous–neurotic dimension. The reason for this is that although life events are common in this disorder, they are not uncommon as triggers of bipolar and unipolar endogenous states. Age of onset under 40 is correct, but this does not discriminate sharply from bipolar depression. "Insidious onset" is in conflict with the presence of life events, which are often closely and impressively related with the development of depression.

"Chronic course" and "poor response to previous treatment" are both at variance with the greater part of the available evidence. In one of the earliest controlled clinical trials of imipramine (Ball & Kiloh, 1959; Kiloh et al., 1962), the response of patients with neurotic depression was not as favorable as that of patients in endogenous cases. However, imipramine did prove effective in a substantial proportion of the former group of patients. This finding has been confirmed in numerous studies, including the three clinical trials of the Boston–New Haven project (Klerman, 1978; Di Mascio et al., 1979; Rowan et al., 1982), which showed amitriptyline to be effective for the attack of illness and also the prevention of relapse (Rowan et al., 1982).

"Chronic course" is not admissible as a general feature. As tricyclic and monoamine oxidase inhibitor drugs and certain forms of psychotherapy have proved effective, and electroconvulsive therapy has been shown to be of value in a substantial proportion of severe and suicidal cases, it is clear that many patients with neurotic depression can achieve relatively stable remissions in response to appropriate management. After many years of recurrent illness, a chronic course may evolve in a number of cases. But unlike dysthymia, neurotic depression is a recurrent (rather than a chronic) illness albeit in the setting of a personality maladjusted to a varying extent in a proportion of cases.

As far as family history is concerned, in light of findings of most authoritative genetic studies (Zimmerman et al., 1986) and the best known twin investigation (Slater, 1953), there appears to be no significant genetic contribution to the etiology of neurotic depression. This is one of the most impressive discriminating features from unipolar disorder proper and its significance is further discussed later.

Certain depressive features are conspicuous by their absence. Psychomotor retardation proves to have the highest weighting among the discriminating factors in an early study that employed multivariate techniques (Carney et al., 1965), and further evidence for its diagnostic value has been adduced by the studies of Parker et al. (1990) and Widlocher (1987). Its presence was consistent with an endogenous form of illness. Absence of psychomotor retardation should therefore receive mention among the criteria. Other useful criteria are *absence* of a "distinct quality" to the depression, and the *presence* of reactivity in the sense of responsiveness to changing circumstances and important life events, favorable or otherwise. A history of previous *episodes* should figure in the clinical profile. A modified version of the clinical profile described by Bronisch and Klerman (1988) derived from this review is shown in Table 8.1.

Reanalysis of the Data from Which Lewis Developed His Unitary Concept of the Affective Disorders

Perhaps the most conclusive body of evidence adduced against the unitary concept of affective disorder formulated by Lewis in 1937 emerged from the anlysis by Kiloh and Garside (1977) of the clinical features described in detail in each of the cases included by Lewis in the three papers he published in the *Journal of Mental Science* (Lewis, 1934a, 1934b, 1936). Each of the principal component analyses of the clinical items (cited in full in Kiloh and Garside's paper) yielded bimodal distributions. When the items of the components were ranked by their numerical weights, they clearly contrasted the features of typical endogenous (or unipolar depression) on the one hand with those recognizable as belonging to the neurotic depressive clinical profile on the other. Cluster analyses yielded identical results.

There were two clusters comprising patients who mainly fell into the (positive) endogenous modes and clusters and those who fell into the neurotic parts of the distributions. There was little overlap. The distribution of principal component scores and of first component scores by cluster were highly significantly non-unimodal. Kiloh and Garside's conclusion was stated as follows: "It appears from the data that endogenous depression is an endogenous condition; patients either have it or do not have it, although of course it may vary in severity." The corollary was that those with neurotic depression were a distinct group that overlapped only by a small margin with the endogenous depressives in relation to the issues discussed here. The literature on this subject has been reviewed in a recent paper (Roth & Caetano, 1995).

The Impact of Eliminating Neurotic Depression

To fully estimate the effects of eliminating neurotic depression from DSM-IV and also from ICD-10, they have to be considered in conjunction with closely related changes in each classification—the deletion of unipolar disorder and the substitution of major depression in DSM-IV and depressive episode together with recurrent depressive episode in ICD-10. When Leonhard (1957) first advanced the concept of the unipolar–bipolar dichotomy, he confined it to endogenous forms of affective disorder. In accordance with a tradition that stems from Kraepelin in European psychiatry, he judged unipolar depression to be distinguished with relative sharpness from neurotic depression. The creators of DSM-III rejected this distinction and amalgamated unipolar disorder with neurotic depression to create the syndrome of major depressive episode (usually recurrent), perhaps the commonest single diagnosis made in psychiatric clinical practice. It is clear from the history of the subject as reviewed by Bronisch and Klerman (1988) that major depression in a hybrid disorder consisted of these two components. The implication of this amalgamation requires review in light of a number of recent inquiries.

It has become increasingly evident from studies conducted during the past 10 to 15 years that unipolar depression is the most common form of affective disorder in first-degree relatives of probands with bipolar depressive illness (Gershon, 1989). The view that a substantial proportion of these unipolar cases probably have a close biological kinship with bipolar affective disorders is supported by other findings (Angst, 1978; Angst et al., 1978, 1979; Zimmerman et al., 1986).

Unipolar patients with an early age of onset, high frequency of episodes, and a family history of bipolar illness have been described by Akiskal et al. (1989) as pseudo-unipolar. Furthermore, Akiskal et al. (1989) and Cassano et al. (1989) reported that these patients are liable to develop hypomanic episodes in the course of treatment with antidepressants. These investigators described patients with the characteristics mentioned earlier as bipolar III, but they have also been designated as unipolar II.

Responsiveness to treatment with lithium provides further evidence for the kinship of the unipolar with bipolar disorders (Goodwin & Jamison, 1990). Unipolar patients whose cyclical depressions are separated by intervals of 12 and 24 months respond to prophylactic treatment with lithium in a similar manner to bipolar patients. There is evidence also that those with florid and severe recurrent attacks of unipolar illness have an affinity to the bipolar group of patients. A growing body of investigators have concluded that the evidence points to the validity of the original Kraepelinian concept which postulated the unity of unipolar and bipolar disorders (Goodwin & Jamison, 1990; Cassano et al., 1992; Akiskal et al., 1989). Indeed, Akiskal earlier subsumed all such patients under a broad bipolar spectrum (Akiskal, 1983).

In light of these findings, unipolar and bipolar depression can be conceived as a closely related group of disorders overlapping in their clinical features and genetic origins and similar in their treatment responses. They can be conceived of as a well-defined endogenous group of disorders in the sense of having a specific genetic basis, characteristic course, and response to treatment suggestive of a specific biological foundation.

Neurotic depression is differentiated from unipolar and bipolar disorders by virtue of its distinctive clinical profile and *irregularly* recurrent course and on the basis of the most authoritative evidence of the absence of any significant hereditary contribution to its causation. It is on a lower hierarchical level than endogenous states in the classification of affective disorders. A disorder with this clinical and genetic profile is not to be found in DSM-III-R and DSM-IV. Its place has been taken in this classification by dysthymia, and neurotic depression is described as synonymous in both DSM-III-R and ICD-10. For reasons that have been argued in this chapter, dysthymia is a different concept and does not replace neurotic depression.

If the thesis developed in this chapter is accepted, major depressive disorder as presently conceived constitutes a mixture of two distinct conditions: unipolar depression and neurotic depression, no matter which name is chosen for the latter disorder.

This concept is likely to cause obfuscation and confusion both in scientific research and in clinical practice in relation to disorders of affect. Unipolar disorder is far more common than bipolar illness. Any neurobiological variables that characterize unipolar depression, including genetic, neurochemical, and endocrine changes that have not yet come to light. On the basis of this review, they may escape detection in the course of investigations of major depressive disorder undertaken with the aid of sound hypotheses and precise scientific techniques. But the view that neurotic depression is identical to unipolar depression is erroneous. It subsumes at least two distinct disorders and probably severe forms of anxiety disorder and other neuroses in addition to neurotic depression. A depressive coloring is ubiquitous in a proportion of all neuroses in their severe forms. This may be one reason for the relative weakness of major depression as a nosological concept according to a number of psychiatrists in different parts of the world (Strömgren, 1983; Roth, 1983).

Further research is needed to resolve many problems that have arisen in recent years in the classification and diagnosis of the unipolar, neurotic, and related forms of affective disorders that have been reviewed in this chapter. Comparative studies are needed in fresh cohorts of patients diagnosed according to the criteria set out here as suffering from (1) neurotic depression, (2) dysthymia, and (3) unipolar depression. The DSM-III criteria should be employed for dysthymia. Those diagnosed as unipolar depression should satisfy criteria for endogenous disorder without evidence of spontaneous or treatment-evoked bouts of hypomania or any form of sustained elation (2 weeks or longer). Unless clinical features similar to those in the depressive swings of bipolar cases are stipulated as diagnostic, unipolar depression is devoid of meaning. Patients should be allocated to the group of neurotic depressions on the basis of the criteria listed here which would need to be more strictly operationalized for purposes of an inquiry.

The presenting clinical features and the personality and developmental background of the three groups should be compared. Their course and outcome need to be investigated over a period of 3 to 4 years to evaluate the stability of the initial diagnoses. In subsamples of patients taken from each group, clinical trials with antidepressant medication and psychological methods of treatment should be undertaken. This is the bare outline of inquiries that would need to be stringently designed in all their aspects.

It is of vital importance for psychiatry that more light should be shed on this area. The disorders listed account for a high proportion of patients treated in inpatient and outpatient psychiatric practice. The scientific weaknesses of major depressive disorder as in DSM-III, which incorporates both unipolar depression and neurotic depression, have already been described. But there are wider pragmatic and philosophical considerations to be taken into account in any review of the taxonomic and other problems they pose. The concept of major depression implicit in a high proportion of contemporary publications in relation to the diagnosis of treatment of major depressive disorder postulates a medical illness in which the predominant causes are hereditary and other biological factors. Examination focuses on the presenting features of the mental state, and the decisions that emerge are expressed in terms of an Axis I diagnosis alone. Developmental and biographical data, adjustment, and personality setting rarely receive mention. In certain forms of inquiry, such as double-blind controlled trials, this exclusive focus is perhaps justifiable, although some of the glaring inconsistencies in the results may stem from failure to control for other variables.

However, it is in neurotic depression and related disorders that a number of psychological treatments have achieved their greatest successes. This point is well exemplified by interpersonal psychotherapy (Klerman et al., 1984) and cognitive psychotherapy (Beck, 1967). The claims in relation to endogenous forms of depression have been much more modest. But in all forms of psychological treatment exploration of the patient's development, previous adjustment, and personality structure is essential. The understanding of the patient that flows from such explorations is of central importance to the practice of psychiatry. Such an understanding also influences the manner in which the professional identity of the psychiatrist is defined by the world outside the clinic. The definition of psychiatrists as doctors who treat mental illness with medication alone is far too often heard from intelligent members of the lay public nowadays. This is a very narrow view of what psychiatrists do. If they are to provide adequate treatment for the group of patients within major depression who were previously diagnosed with neurotic depression, psychiatrists must make sensitive responses and listen, support, empathize, and understand patients as well as provide needed medication. Psychiatrists should have the requisite range of training, knowledge, and experience required to encompass and manage the disorders of cerebral and mental functioning and the biological, psychological, and social dimensions of illness in this area. Neurotic depression is a paradigm of this group of conditions. Our knowledge of its origins is dwarfed by our ignorance, but imaginative scientific response to its challenges by multidisciplinary teams can be expected to yield fresh findings that will shed light in many of the dark places within psychiatry.

"Personal depression" has much to commend it as an alternative to neurotic depression. The depressed mood and state of those with neurotic depression can almost invariably be traced through *some lines* of continuity to personality features or difficulties; these do not necessarily merit a diagnosis of personality disorder.

The long-term follow-up study of Andrews et al. (1990) provides further factual validation for personal depression as an appropriate designation for the syndrome of neurotic depression. In endogenous depression personality factors accounted for only 2% of variance in respect to outcome. In neurotic depression, these factors explained 20% of the variance. In a review of the differentiation of anxiety and depressive disorders in an earlier section of this chapter, data were quoted that suggest that further exploration of the developmental history, adjustment, and premorbid personality profile of neurotic patients might yield findings that permit better prediction of the fate of those with personal or neurotic depression, as well as those with anxiety disorder.

References

Akiskal, H. S. (1983). The bipolar spectrum: New concepts in classification and diagnosis. In L. Grinspoon (Ed.), *Psychiatry update: The American Psychiatric Association annual review* (Vol. 2, pp. 271–292). Washington, DC: American Psychiatric Press.

Akiskal, H. S. (1990). Towards a definition of dysthymia: Boundaries with personality and mood disorders. In S. W. Burton & H. S. Akiskal (Eds.), *Dysthymic disorder* (pp. 1–12). London: Gaskell.

Akiskal, H. S., Bitar, A. H., Puzantian, V. R., Rosenthal, T. L., & Walker, P. W. (1978). The nosological status of neurotic depression. *Archives of General Psychiatry, 136*, 57–61.

Akiskal, H. S., Cassano, G. B., Musetti, L., Perugi, G., Tundo, A., & Mignani, V. (1989). Psychopathology, temperament, and past course in primary major depressions: I. Review of evidence for a bipolar spectrum. *Psychopathology, 22*, 268–277.

Akiskal, H. S., Rosenthal, R. H., Rosenthal, T. L., Kashgarian, M., Khani, M. K., & Puzantian, V. R. (1979). Differentiation of primary affective illness from situational, symptomatic and secondary depressions. *Archives of General Psychiatry, 36*, 653–643.

American Psychiatric Association. (1968). *Diagnostic and statistical manual of mental disorders* (2nd ed.). Washington, DC: Author.

American Psychiatric Association. (1980). *Diagnostic and statistical manual of mental disorders* (3rd ed.). Washington, DC: Author.

American Psychiatric Association. (1987). *Diagnostic and statistical manual of mental disorders* (3rd ed., rev.). Washington, DC: Author.

American Psychiatric Association. (1994). *Diagnostic and statistical manual of mental disorders* (4th ed.). Washington, DC: Author.

Andrews, G., Stewart, G., Morris-Yates, A., Holt, P., & Henderson, S. (1990). Evidence for a general neurotic syndrome. *British Journal of Psychiatry, 157*, 6–12.

Angst, J. (1978). The course of affective disorders: II. Typology of bipolar manic–depressive illness. *Archiv für Psychiatrie und Nervenkrankheiten, 226*, 65–73.

Angst, J., Felder, W., & Frey, R. (1979). The course of unipolar and bipolar affective disorders. In M. Schou & E. Stromgren (Eds.), *Origin, prevention and treatment of affective disorder* (pp. 215–226). London: Academic Press.

Angst, J., Felder, W., Frey, R., & Stassen, H. H. (1978). The course of affective disorders: I. Change of diagnosis of monopolar, unipolar and bipolar illness. *Archiv für Psychiatrie und Nervenkrankheiten, 226*, 57–64.

Ball, J. R. B., & Kiloh, L. G. (1959). A controlled trial of imipramine in treatment of depressive states. *British Medical Journal, 2*, 1052–1055.

Barraclough, B., Bunch, J., Nelson, B., & Sainsbury, P. (1974). A hundred cases of suicide: Clinical aspects. *British Journal of Psychiatry, 125*, 355–373.

Beck, A. T. (1967). *Depression: Causes and treatment.* Philadelphia: University of Pennsylvania Press.

Bronisch, T., & Klerman, G. L. (1988). The current status of neurotic depression as a diagnostic category. *Psychiatric Developments, 64*, 245–276.

Bronisch, T., Wittchen, H. U., Krieg, C. H., Rupp, H. U., & von Zerssen, D. (1985). Depressive neurosis: A long-term prospective and retrospective follow-up of former inpatients. *Acta Psychiatrica Scandinavica, 71*, 237–248.

Carney, M. W. P., Roth, M., & Garside, R. F. (1965). The diagnosis of depressive syndromes and the prediction of ECT response. *British Journal of Psychiatry, 111*, 659–674.

Cassano, G. B., Akiskal, H. S., Savino, M., Musetti, L., Perugi, G., & Soriani, A. (1992). Proposed subtypes of bipolar II and related disorders: With hypomanic episodes (or cyclothymia) and with hyperthymic temperament. *Journal of Affective Disorders, 26*, 127–140.

Di Mascio, A., Weissman, M. M., Prusoff, B. A., Neu, C., Zwilling, M., & Klerman, G. L. (1979). Differential symptom reduction by drugs and psychotherapy in acute depression. *Archives of General Psychiatry, 36*, 1450–1456.

Eysenck, H. M. (1959). *Manual of the Maudsley Personality Inventory.* London: London University Press.

Falide, M., Eisemann, M., & Perris, C. (1987). Psychiatric morbidity among relatives of different subgroups of neurotic depression. *Acta Psychiatrica Scandinavica, 75*, 487–490.

Garside, R. F., Kay, D. W. K., Wilson, I. C., Deaton, I. D., & Roth, M. (1971). Depressive syndromes and classification of patients. *Psychological Medicine, 1,* 333–338.

Gershon, E. S. (1989). Recent developments in genetics of manic–depressive illness. *Journal of Clinical Psychiatry, 50,* 4–7.

Goldin, L. R., & Gershon, E. S. (1988). The genetic epidemiology of major depressive illness. In A. J. Frances & R. E. Hales (Eds.), *Review of psychiatry* (Vol. 7, pp. 149–168). Washington, DC: American Psychiatric Press.

Goodwin, F. K., & Jamison, K. R. (1990). *Manic–depressive illness.* New York: Oxford University Press.

Grinker, R. R., Miller, J., Sabshin, M., Nunn, R., & Nunnally, J. C. (1961). *The phenomenon of depression.* New York: Harper & Row.

Gurney, C., Roth, M., Garside, R. F., Kerr, T. A., & Schapira, K. (1972). Studies in the classification of affective disorders. The relationship between anxiety states and depressive illnesses. II. *British Journal of Psychiatry, 121,* 162–166.

Hickie, I., Parsonage, B., & Parker, G. (1990). Prediction of response to electroconvulsive therapy. *British Journal of Psychiatry, 157,* 65–71.

Hirschfeld, R. M. A. (1990). Personality and dysthymia. In S. W. Burton & H. S. Akiskal (Eds.), *Dysthymic disorder* (pp. 69–77). London: Gaskell.

Kay, D. W. K., Garside, R. F., Roy, J. R., & Beamish, P. (1969). Endogenous and neurotic syndromes of depression: A 40-year follow-up of 104 cases. *British Journal of Psychiatry, 115,* 389–399.

Kendell, R. E. (1968). *The classification of depressive illness* (Maudsley Monograph No. 18). London: Institute of Psychiatry, Oxford University Press.

Kendell, R. E., & Gourlay, J. (1970). The clinical distinction between psychotic and neurotic depressions. *British Journal of Psychiatry, 117,* 257–266.

Kerr, T. A., Roth, M., & Schapira, K. (1974). The prediction of outcome of anxiety states and depressive illnesses. *British Journal of Psychiatry, 124,* 125–133.

Kerr, T. A., Roth, M., Schapira, K., & Gurney, C. (1972). The assessment of prediction of outcome in affective disorders. *British Journal of Psychiatry, 21,* 167–174.

Kiloh, L. G., Andrews, G., & Neilson, R. M. (1988). The long-term outcome of depressive illness. *British Journal of Psychiatry, 153,* 752–757.

Kiloh, L. G., Andrews, G., Neilson, M., & Bianchi, G. N. (1972). The relationship of syndromes called endogenous and neurotic depression. *British Journal of Psychiatry, 121,* 183–196.

Kiloh, L. G., & Ball, J. R. B. (1961). Depression treated with imipramine: A follow-up study. *British Medical Journal, 1,* 168–171.

Kiloh, L. G., Ball, J. R. B., & Garside, R. F. (1962). Prognostic factors in the treatment of depressive states with imipramine. *British Medical Journal, 1,* 1225–1227.

Kiloh, L. G., & Garside, R. F. (1963). The independence of neurotic depression and endogenous depression. *British Journal of Psychiatry, 109,* 451–463.

Kiloh, L. G., & Garside, R. F. (1977). Original articles—depression: A multivariate study of Sir Aubrey Lewis's data on melancholia. *Australian and New Zealand Journal of Psychiatry, 11,* 149–156.

Klein, D., & Davis, J. (1969). *Diagnosis and drug treatment of psychiatric disorders* (pp. 180–185). Baltimore: Williams & Wilkins.

Klerman, G. L. (1978). Combining drugs and psychotherapy in the treatment of depression. In J. O. Cole, A. F. Schatzberg, & S. H. Frazier (Eds.), *Depression: Biology, psychodynamics and treatment* (pp. 213–227). New York: Plenum Press.

Klerman, G. L. (1986). Scientific status of neurotic depression. *Psychopathology, 18,* 163–173.

Klerman, G. L., Endicott, J., Spitzer, R., & Hirschfeld, R. M. A. (1979). Neurotic depressions: A systematic analysis of multiple criteria and meanings. *American Journal of Psychiatry, 136,* 57–61.

Klerman, G. L., Weissman, M. M., Rounsaville, B. J., & Chevron, E. S. (1984). *Interpersonal psychotherapy of depression.* New York: Basic Books.

Kraepelin, E. (1921). *Manic–depressive insanity and paranoia* (R. M. Barclay, Trans.; G. M. Robertson, Ed.). Edinburgh: Livingstone.

Kraepelin, E. (1986). *Ein Lehrbuch für Studirende und Aerzte* (8th ed.). Leipzig: J. A. Barth. (Original work published 1913)

Lazare, A., & Klerman, G. (1968). Hysteria and depression: The frequency and significance hysterical personality in hospitalized depressed women. *American Journal of Psychiatry, 124*(Suppl. 11), 48–56.

Leonhard, K. (1957). *Aufteilung der Endogenen Psychosen.* Berlln Akademie Verlag.

Lewis, A. J. (1934a). Melancholia: A historical review. *Journal of Mental Science, 80,* 1–42.

Lewis, A. J. (1934b). Melancholia: A clinical survey of depressive states. *Journal of Mental Science, 80,* 277–378.

Lewis, A. J. (1936). Melancholia: Prognostic studies and case material. *Journal of Mental Science, 82,* 488–558.

Lorr, M., Pokorny, A. D., & Klett, C. J. (1973). Three depressive types. *Journal of Clinical Psychology, 29,* 290–294.

Matussek, P., Soeldner, M., & Nagel, D. (1982). Neurotic depression results of cluster analyses. *Journal of Nervous and Mental Disease, 170,* 588–597.

Mendels, J., & Cochrane, C. (1968). The nosology of depression: The endogenous-reactive concept. *American Journal of Psychiatry, 124*(Suppl.), 1–11.

Mountjoy, C. Q., & Roth, M. (1982a). Studies in the relationship between depressive disorders and anxiety states: I. Rating scales. *Journal of Affective Disorders, 4,* 127–147.

Mountjoy, C. Q., & Roth, M. (1982b). Studies in the relationship between depressive disorders and anxiety states: II. Clinical items. *Journal of Affective Disorders, 4,* 148–161.

Nemiah, J. C. (1975). Depressive neurosis. In A. M. Freedman, H. Kaplan, & B. J. Sadock (Eds.), *Comprehensive textbook of psychiatry* (2nd ed., Vol. 1, pp. 1255–1264). Baltimore: Williams & Wilkins.

Ni Bhrolchain, M., Brown, G. W., & Harris, T. O. (1979). Psychotic and neurotic depression: 2. Clinical characteristics. *British Journal of Psychiatry, 134,* 94–107.

Overall, J. E., Hollister, L. E., & Johnson, M. (1966). Nosology of depression and differential response to drugs. *Journal of the American Medical Association, 195,* 946–950.

Parker, G., Hadzi-Pavlovic, D., Boyce, P., Wilhelm, K., Brodaty, H., Mitchell, P., Hickie, I., & Eyers, K. (1990). Classifying depression by mental state signs. *British Journal of Psychiatry, 157,* 55–65.

Paykel, E. S. (1971). Classification of depressed patients. A cluster analysis derived for grouping. *British Journal of Psychiatry, 118,* 265–288.

Paykel, E. S. (1972). Typologies and response to amitriptyline. *British Journal of Psychiatry, 120,* 147–156.

Pilowsky, J., Levine, S., & Boulton, D. M. (1969). The classification of depression by numerical taxonomy. *British Journal of Psychiatry, 115,* 937–945.

Post, R. M., Rubinow, D. R., & Balleneger, J. C. (1984). Conditioning, sensitization and kindling: Implications for the course of affective illness. In R. M. Post & J. C. Ballenger (Eds.), *The neurobiology of mood disorders* (pp. 432–466). Baltimore: Williams & Wilkins.

Raskin, A., & Crook, T. H. (1976). The endogenous–neurotic distinction as a predictor of response to antidepressant drugs. *Psychological Medicine, 6,* 59–70.

Riskind, J. H., Beck, A. T., Berchick, R. J., Brown, G. & Steer, R. A. (1987). Reliability of DSM-III diagnoses for major depression and generalized anxiety disorder using the structured clinical interview for DSM-III. *Archives of General Psychiatry, 44,* 817–820.

Rosenthal, S. H., & Klerman, G. L. (1966). Content and consistency in the endogenous depressive pattern. *British Journal of Psychiatry, 112,* 471–484.

Rosenthal, S. H., & Gudeman, J. E. (1967). The endogenous depressive pattern: An empirical investigation. *Archives of General Psychiatry, 16,* 241–249.

Roth, M. (1977). The borderlands of anxiety and depressive states and their bearing on new and old models for the classification of depression. In H. M. Van Praag & J. Bruinvels (Eds.), *Neuro-transmission and disturbed behaviour* (pp. 109–157). Utrecht: Scheltema-Holkema.

Roth, M. (1978). The classification of affective disorders. *Pharmacopsychiatria, 11,* 27–42.

Roth, M. (1979). A new classification of the affective disorders. In B. Saletu et al. (Eds.), *Neuropsychopharmacology* (pp. 255–273). New York: Pergamon Press.

Roth, M. (1983). The achievements and limitations of DSM-III. In R. L. Spitzer, J. B. W. Williams, & A. E. Skodol (Eds.), *International perspectives on DSM-III* (pp. 91–105). Washington, DC: American Psychiatric Press.

Roth, M. (1984). Agoraphobia, panic disorder and generalized anxiety disorder: Some implications of recent advances. *Psychiatric Developments, 2,* 31–52.

Roth, M., & Barnes, T. R. E. (1981). The classification of affective disorders: A synthesis of old and new concepts. *Comprehensive Psychiatry, 22,* 54–77.

Roth, M., & Caetano, D. (1995). Classification of the affective and related disorders. In M. Ackenheil, B. Bondy, R. Engel, M. Ermann, & N. Nedopil (Eds.), *Implications of psychopharmacology to psychiatry: Biological, nosological, and therapeutical concepts* (pp. 101–126). Heidelberg: Springer.

Roth, M., Gurney, C., Garside, R. F., Kerr, T. A., & Schapira, K. (1972). Studies in the classification of affective disorders: The relationship between anxiety states and depressive illness. *British Journal of Psychiatry, 121,* 147–161.

Roth, M., & Mountjoy, C. Q. (1982). The distinction between anxiety states and depressive disorders. In E. S. Paykel (Ed.), *Handbook of affective disorders* (pp. 70–92). London: Churchill Livingstone.

Roth, M., & Mountjoy, C. Q. (1992). The relationship between anxiety and depressive disorders. In D. J. Kupfer (Ed.), *Reflections on modern psychiatry* (pp. 9–24). Washington, DC: American Psychiatric Press.

Rowan, P. R., Paykel, E. S., & Parker, R. R. (1982). Phenelzine, amitriptyline: Effects on symptoms of neurotic depression. *British Journal of Psychiatry, 140,* 475–483.

Roy, A., Sutton, M., & Pickar, D. (1985). Neuroendocrine and personality variables in dysthymic disorder. *American Journal of Psychiatry, 142,* 94–97.

Schapira, K., Roth, M., Kerr, T. A., & Gurney, C. (1972). The prognosis of affective disorders. The differentiation of anxiety states from depressive illness. *British Journal of Psychiatry, 121,* 165–181.

Sieveright, N., & Tyrer, P. (1990). Relationship of dysthymia to anxiety and other neurotic disorders. In S. W. Burton & H. S. Akiskal (Eds.), *Dysthymic disorder* (pp. 24–36). London: Gaskell.

Slater, E. (1943). The neurotic constitution: A statistical study of two thousand neurotic soldiers. *Journal of Neurology and Psychiatry, 6,* 1–16.

Slater, E. (1953). Psychotic and neurotic illness in twins. *Special Report Series of the Medical Research Council,* No. 278.

Slater, E., & Roth, M. (1977). *Clinical psychiatry.* London: Bailliere, Tindall & Cassell.

Slater, E., & Shields, J. (1969). Genetical aspects of anxiety. *British Journal of Psychiatry, 3,* 62–71.

Spitzer, R. L., Endicott, J., & Robins, E. (1978). Research diagnostic criteria: Rationale and reliability. *Archives of General Psychiatry, 35,* 773–782.

Spitzer, R., & Sheehy, M. (1976). DSM-III: A classification system in treatment. *Psychiatric Annals, 6,* 102–109.

Strömgren, E. (1983). The strengths and weaknesses of DSM-III. In R. L. Spitzer, J. B. W. Williams, & A. E. Skodol (Eds.), *International perspectives on DSM-III* (pp. 69–78). Washington, DC: American Psychiatric Press.

Tellenbach, H. (1976). *Melancholie.* Berlin Springer-Verlag.

Torgersen, S. (1983). Genetic factors in anxiety disorders. *Archives of General Psychiatry, 40,* 1085–1089.

Torgersen, S. (1986). Genetic factors in moderately severe and mild affective disorders. *Archives of General Psychiatry, 43,* 222–226.

Tyrer, P. (1989). *Classification of neurosis.* New York: Wiley.

von Zerssen, D. (1982). Personality and affective disorders. In E. S. Paykel (Ed.), *Handbook of affective disorders* (pp. 214–228). Edinburgh: Churchill Livingstone.

Widlocher, D. (1987). Inhibition and depression. In K. Biziere, S. Garattini, & P. Simon (Eds.), *Quo vadis? Diagnosis and treatment of depression* (pp. 73–89). Montpellier: Sanofi Recherche.

Winokur, G. (1985). The validity of neurotic–reactive depression. *Archives of General Psychiatry, 42,* 116–1122.

World Health Organization. (1992). *The ICD-10 classification of mental and behavioural disorders: Clinical descriptions and diagnositic guidelines.* Geneva: Author.

Zimmerman, M. M., Coryell, W., & Pfhol, B. (1986). Validity of familial subtypes of primary unipolar depression. Clinical demographic, and psychosocial correlates. *Archives of General Psychiatry, 43,* 1090–1096.

Zimmerman, M. M., Coryell, W., Pfohl, B., & Stangl, D. D. (1987). An American validation study of the Newcastle Diagnostic Scale: II. Relationship with clinical, demographic, familial and psychosocial features. *British Journal of Psychiatry, 150,* 526–532.

CHAPTER 9

A Critical Reappraisal of the Concept of Neurotic Depression

Mario Maj

Neurotic depression remains, especially in some European countries, a popular diagnostic concept.

Actually, not all psychiatrists, at least in Europe, are aware of the innovations brought about by DSM-III (American Psychiatric Association, 1980) and its successors in the nomenclature and classification of mental disorders, and, among those who have been able to appreciate them, several have regarded them as irrelevant to their professional practice, for one or more of the following reasons: (1) They consider classificatory matters a non-essential aspect of psychiatric work; (2) they are skeptical about every diagnostic novelty (for them, who have been seeing patients for so many years, there may be nothing really new); (3) they believe that diagnostic manuals are research instruments, which are not expected to be used in clinical routine; (4) they believe that DSM-III and its successors reflect a biologically oriented approach that has been carried to clinically unacceptable extreme; (5) they regard DSM as a system tailored for use in hospitalized patients and unsuitable for application in ambulatory settings; (6) they are convinced that DSM reflects American diagnostic habits, and that it is appropriate for non-American psychiatrists to adopt the *International Classification of Diseases* (ICD); and (7) they are persuaded that the classification proposed in the DSM-III and its successors is inaccurate and/or does not fit clinical reality.

All these sources of "resistance" have been certainly working in favor of the survival of the concept of neurotic depression, because this concept is deeply rooted in clinical practice (especially that of psychodynamically oriented psychiatrists working in ambulatory settings), has a long tradition in the European psychiatric literature, and was included in ICD-9 (World Health Organization, 1978) (which was in force until 1992).

The survival of the concept of neurotic depression in clinical usage and some recent proposals to revive it in official classifications are reasons for a critical reappraisal. This chapter includes a brief overview of the concept, an analysis of the reasons why it was dismissed from the most recent diagnostic systems, an outline of the diagnostic categories that have replaced it, a survey of the latest attempts to revive it, and a discussion of future perspectives.

Overview of the Concept of Neurotic Depression

In both ICD-8 (World Health Organization, 1974) and ICD-9 (World Health Organization, 1978), neurotic depression was defined by the following elements: (1) onset preceded by a stressful event, (2) intensity of depression out of proportion to the event, (3) absence of delusions and hallucinations, (4) connection between the depressive themes and the precipitating event, (5) presence of anxiety, (6) nonsevere degree of mood disturbance, (7) presence of "other neurotic characteristics" (conceivably, the "hysterical symptoms, phobias, obsessional and compulsive symptoms" listed in the general definition of neurotic disorders), (8) absence of "other psychotic characteristics" (conceivably, the "perplexity, disturbed attitude to self, disorder of perception and behavior" mentioned, besides delusions and hallucinations, in the general definition of affective psychoses), (9) unimpaired reality testing, (10) socially acceptable behavior and not disorganized personality, and (11) no demonstrable organic basis.

Psychodynamic mechanisms were invoked by the DSM-II (American Psychiatric Association, 1968) definition of depressive neurosis ("an excessive reaction of depression due to an internal conflict or to an identifiable event") and, above all, in the general definition of neuroses provided in that classification (disorders in which the "chief characteristic" is anxiety whether "felt and expressed directly" or "controlled unconsciously and automatically by conversion, displacement and various other psychological mechanisms").

This intrusion of psychoanalytic concepts in the clinical characterization of the disorder was not unusual in the European and American literature of the 1960s and 1970s. As late as 1982, the influential clinician and clinical psychopharmacologist Paul Kielholz opened the chapter "Neurotic Depressions" in his booklet *Masked Depression* (Kielholz et al., 1982) with the following sentences:

At the origin of neurotic depressions are conflict situations dating back to early childhood (such as separation from the mother during infancy, an atmosphere of tension in the home, or a disturbed child-parent relationship), which the patient has been unable to abreact, which he has failed to cope with satisfactorily, or which he has partially or completely repressed.

Such unconscious processes of repression constitute a permanent potential source of trouble, which may later, e.g., in situations of tension or during biologically critical phases of life, manifest itself in the form of a depressive state. (p. 25)

The foregoing considerations would perhaps suggest that neurotic depression was consistently regarded as qualitatively different from manic–depressive psychosis, depressed type (inclusion terms: depressive psychosis, endogenous depression, psychotic depression) (ICD-9; World Health Organization, 1978) from both the symptomatological and the etiopathogenetic viewpoints. This, however, was not actually the case. As reviewed by Kendell (1976), neurotic–reactive and psychotic–endogenous depression were alternatively characterized, in the psychiatric literature of the 1960s and 1970s, in five different ways: (1) as distinct illnesses; (2) as two variants, the former mild and chronic and the latter severe and acute, of a single illness; (3) as poles of a psychotic–neurotic continuum; (4) as extremes of a continuous distribution portrayed by two orthogonal dimensions (psychotic and neurotic); and (5) as hierarchically related conditions (neurotic depression being diagnosed when the characteristic features of endogenous depression are lacking).

The "dichotomous" view (regarding neurotic and endogenous depression as distinct illnesses) was especially upheld by the Newcastle group. In a multiple regression analysis performed on the clinical ratings of a population of depressed inpatients, diagnosed clinically as endogenous or neurotic, that distinguished group found that the distribution of the scores on the resulting function was bimodal (Carney et al., 1965). Consistent findings were obtained by the Harvard group (Rosenthal & Gudeman, 1967) in a factor analysis study of acutely depressed women: after a first factor corresponding to the endogenous or "autonomous" pattern, a second one was produced, with a symptom pattern consisting of hypochondriasis, psychic anxiety, demanding and complaining behavior, self-pity and blaming the environment, and somatic anxiety ("self-pitying constellation"). The scores of this second pattern correlated positively with the presence of apparent precipitants prior to the onset of symptoms and with anxious–neurasthenic personality traits, and negatively with a history of previous episodes requiring hospitalization.

Subsequent studies based on factor or cluster analysis, however, although almost consistently producing a factor or cluster corresponding to the endogenous pattern, did not, by and large, generate a factor or cluster identifiable with neurotic depression, thus justifying the view that "psychotic or endogenous depression is a condition with a restricted range of clinical manifestations, consistent with an imputed genetic or biochemical basis, whilst so-called neurotic depression is a diffuse entity encompassing some of the ways in which the patient utilizes his defense mechanisms to cope with his own neuroticism and concurrent environmental stress" (Kiloh et al., 1972, p. 194).

Reasons for the Dismissal of Neurotic Depression from Recent Diagnostic Systems

The reviewed evidence from factor and cluster analysis studies, suggesting that the concept of endogenous depression is "more soundly based" than that of neurotic depression (Kendell, 1976), was reinforced by Spitzer and Wilson's (1975) report of a very low agreement among clinicians in the diagnosis of neurotic depression (interrater reliability coefficient of .37). Subsequently, two influential papers (Akiskal et al., 1978; Klerman et al., 1979) virtually sanctioned the exclusion of the category of neurotic depression from the upcoming DSM-III.

In the first, Akiskal et al. (1978) reported on a 3- to 4-year prospective follow-up of 100 patients whose index episode fulfilled DSM-II (American Psychiatric Association, 1968) criteria for depressive neurosis. Of them, 40 received a follow-up diagnosis of primary affective disorder according to Feighner's (Feighner et al., 1972) criteria (28 had endogenous and 10 had psychotic depressive episodes, whereas 18 had also manic or hypomanic episodes); 38 were found to suffer from nonaffective psychiatric disorders whose exacerbations and remissions were accompanied by oscillations of a depressive symptomatology, usually mild; 10 were found to have a medical or surgical illness on which depression was superimposed; 10 had a prolonged intermittent depressive syndrome but did not fulfill Feighner's criteria for any psychiatric disorder; 2 remained symptom-free throughout the follow-up period. The conclusion was that the concept of neurotic depression encompasses a heterogeneous group of disorders and, therefore, is not clinically meaningful.

In the latter study, Klerman et al. (1979) selected 93 patients meeting Research Diagnostic Criteria (RDC; Spitzer et al., 1975) for major depression, and classified them according to some RDC subtypes relevant to the concept of neurotic depression (i.e., endogenous–nonendogenous, psychotic–nonpsychotic, socially incapacitating–not incapacitating, situational–nonsituational). Of the 38 patients with a nonendogenous depression, 21% were found to be psychotic, 34% were socially invalidated, and

32% had no clear precipitant, whereas, of the 67 patients with a nonpsychotic depression, 55% were classified as endogenous, 37% were socially invalidated, and 46% did not have a precipitant. Only 16 patients (18%) fulfilled simultaneously the criteria for nonendogenous, nonpsychotic, nonincapacitating, and situational depression. The conclusion was that the concept of neurotic depression has different meanings with only a modest degree of overlap and, therefore, should no longer be used.

Besides the above concerns about the reliability and validity of the concept, the other factors that contributed to the dismissal of neurotic depression from DSM-III (and, even before, from RDC) were the rejection of the term "neurosis" (which "had assumed strongly psychodynamic overtones of etiology") (Skodol & Spitzer, 1983, p. 31) and the evidence that many patients labeled "neurotic" were deprived of maintenance treatment with antidepressants after the acute episode and treated with minor tranquilizers, which favored the development of chronicity (Weissman & Klerman, 1977).

Categories Replacing Neurotic Depression in Recent Diagnostic Systems

Research Diagnostic Criteria

In the RDC, published in 1975, three depressive categories are included: major depressive disorder, episodic minor depressive disorder, and chronic and intermittent minor depressive disorder.

Major depressive disorder is defined by a persistent and relatively prominent dysphoric mood, at least five out of eight symptoms (items 1 to 8 in Table 9.1), and a duration of more than 2 weeks. Criteria are provided for 10 subtypes: primary, secondary, recurrent, psychotic, incapacitating, endogenous, agitated, retarded, situational, and simple.

Episodic minor depressive disorder is characterized by a relatively persistent depressed mood (which may be coequal with anxiety), at least 2 out of 16 symptoms (listed in Table 9.1), and a duration of at least 2 weeks. The patient must not meet the criteria for major depressive disorder or chronic and intermittent minor depressive disorder. A subtype with "significant anxiety" is provided.

The criteria for chronic and intermittent minor depressive disorder require at least 2 years of depressed mood much of the time, accompanied by at least 2 of the 16 symptoms listed in Table 9.1. The patient may have had previous episodes of major depression or episodic minor depression or may later develop major depressive, manic, or hypomanic episodes, in which case both diagnoses should be given.

TABLE 9.1. Symptoms Other than Dysphoric or Depressed Mood Listed in the RDC for Major Depressive Disorder, Episodic Minor Depressive Disorder, and Chronic and Intermittent Minor Depressive Disorder

1. Poor appetite or weight loss, or increased appetite or weight gain
2. Sleep difficulty or sleeping too much
3. Loss of energy, fatigability or tiredness
4. Psychomotor agitation or retardation
5. Loss of interest or pleasure in usual activities
6. Feelings of self-reproach, or excessive or inappropriate guilt
7. Diminished ability to think or concentrate
8. Recurrent thoughts of death or suicide, or any suicidal behavior
*9. Nonverbal manifestations of depression such as tearfulness or sad face
*10. Pessimistic attitude
*11. Brooding about past or current unpleasant events
*12. Preoccupation with feelings of inadequacy
*13. Resentful, irritable, angry, or complaining
*14. Demandingness, or clinging dependency
*15. Self-pity
*16. Excessive somatic concern

Note. Asterisk (*) indicates the symptoms listed only in the definitions of minor depressive disorders.

For the purposes of our discussion, the most significant features of this classification are the following: (1) It is acknowledged that depressive disorders may be either severe or mild, and that the latter may be either episodic or chronic; (2) it is specified that mild depressions may differ from severe ones also qualitatively (out of 16 symptoms listed in the definitions of minor depression, 8 are not shared with major depression, and these last include all the items of the above-mentioned "self-pitying constellation" (Rosenthal & Gudeman, 1967); (3) it is mentioned that in mild depression the depressed mood frequently coexists with prominent anxiety, and the possibility is given to specify the presence of this feature; and (4) it is recognized that mild depression may either be a sequela of major depressive episodes or may precede the development of major depression or mania.

In a general practice study carried out in Great Britain, Paykel (1986) found that patients with a Present State Examination (PSE)/CATEGO (Wing et al., 1974) diagnosis of N+ (neurotic depression) received in 55% of cases an RDC diagnosis of major depressive disorder and in 45% one of minor depressive disorder. In another general practice study conducted in Germany, Winter et al. (1991) discovered that, of 194 patients left with a DSM-III-R (American Psychiatric Association, 1987) diagnosis of depressive disorder not otherwise specified (including 103 subjects with a coexistence of depression and anxiety), 47% fulfilled RDC for minor depressive disorder, and 26% RDC for major depressive disorder. Finally, in a general practice investigation carried out in the United States, Barrett et al. (1988) found that episodic minor depressive disorder was the most common specific RDC diagnosis (3.6% of cases, vs. 2.2% for major depressive disorder and 2.1% for chronic and intermittent minor depressive disorder).

DSM-III

In DSM-III, published in 1980, operational criteria are provided for two depressive categories: major depression and dysthymic disorder. Moreover, a descriptive definition is given for adjustment disorder with depressed mood, and a residual category, "atypical depression," is included.

Major depression is defined by a prominent and relatively persistent dysphoric mood or loss of interest or pleasure in all or almost all usual activities and pastimes, and at least four from a list of eight symptoms almost exactly corresponding to those indicated in the RDC definition of major depressive disorder, each present nearly every day for at least 2 weeks. Criteria are provided for subtypes "with psychotic features" and "with melancholia."

Dysthymic disorder (which carries in brackets the specification "or depressive neurosis") is characterized by a depressive syndrome occupying the past 2 years, persistently or with periods of normal mood of no more than a few months, whose severity and duration do not meet the criteria for major depression. During the depressive periods, there is either prominent depressed mood or marked loss of interest or pleasure in all or almost all usual activities or pastimes, and the patient must have at least 3 out of 13 symptoms (Table 9.2, first column). It is specified that major depression may be superimposed upon dysthymic disorder, and that the latter is particularly common in subjects with borderline, histrionic, and dependent personality disorders.

It is clear that the DSM-III concepts of major depression and dysthymic disorder largely correspond, respectively, to the RDC categories of major depressive disorder and chronic and intermittent minor depressive disorder. No category is left in DSM-III for episodic mild depressions.

In RDC all the symptoms listed in the definition of major depression also appear in that of minor depression; in DSM-III, psychomotor retardation or agitation and appetite disturbances are only mentioned in the criteria for major depression. Moreover, the DSM-III definition of dysthymic disorder does not include the excessive somatic concern and the demandingness or clinging dependence appearing in RDC for minor depressions.

Torgersen (1986), in a study carried out on psychiatric inpatients and outpatients, reported that 49% of those who received an ICD-9 (World

TABLE 9.2. Symptoms Listed in the DSM-III and DSM-III-R Criteria for Dysthymia

DSM-III

1. Insomnia or hypersomnia
2. Low energy level or chronic tiredness
3. Feelings of inadequacy, loss of self-esteem, or self-deprecation
4. Decreased effectiveness or productivity at school, work, or home
5. Decreased attention, concentration, or ability to think clearly
6. Social withdrawal
7. Loss of interest in or enjoyment of pleasurable activities
8. Irritability or excessive anger (in children, expressed toward parents or caretakers)
9. Inability to respond with apparent pleasure to praise or rewards
10. Less active or talkative than usual, or feels slowed down or restless
11. Pessimistic attitude toward the future, brooding about past events, or feeling sorry for self
12. Tearfulness or crying
13. Recurrent thoughts of death or suicide

DSM-III-R

1. Poor appetite or overeating
2. Insomnia or hypersomnia
3. Low energy or fatigue
4. Low self-esteem
5. Poor concentration or difficulty making decisions
6. Feelings of hopelessness

Note. Derived from American Psychiatric Association (1980, 1987).

Health Organization, 1978) diagnosis of neurotic depression were classified as having major depression according to DSM-III, whereas 19% had dysthymic disorder, 19% adjustment disorder with depressed mood, and 1% atypical depression. Perris et al. (1982), in a study conducted on hospitalized psychiatric patients, found that neurotic–reactive depression (diagnosed on the basis of their own criteria [d'Elia, et al., 1974], largely consistent with those of ICD-9) corresponded to the DSM-III categories of major depression (49% of cases), atypical depression (23%), dysthymic disorder (14%), and adjustment disorder with depressed mood (14%). These data indicate that the DSM-III concept of dysthymic disorder is much narrower than that of neurotic depression.

Akiskal (1983; Akiskal et al., 1980) suggested that DSM-III dysthymia is in its turn a heterogeneous entity including four subtypes: (1) a residual low-grade chronic depression following one or more major depressive episodes, (2) a chronic dysphoric syndrome superimposed on long-standing nonaffective psychiatric disorders or incapacitating medical diseases, (3) a subsyndromal variant of primary affective illness (with early onset, frequent family history of unipolar or bipolar affective disorders, presence of anhedonic or hypersomnic-retarded features, frequent decrease of rapid eye movement [REM] sleep latency, and frequent favorable response to tricyclic antidepressants and/or lithium, with possible switch to hypomania under treatment with the former), that can be conceptualized as a "depressive temperament" (Akiskal & Akiskal, 1992) upon which major depressive episodes are often superimposed ("subaffective dysthymia"); and (4) an early onset condition of irritable dysphoria, more frequent in women, seldom complicated by major depressive episodes, in which a "melange of dependent, histrionic and antisocial features" is frequently present, substance abuse and familial alcoholism and sociopathy are common, REM sleep latency is usually normal, and response to tricyclic antidepressants and lithium is commonly poor.

DSM-III-R

In DSM-III-R, published in 1987, depressive categories include major depression, dysthymia (again with the specification in brackets "or depressive neurosis"), adjustment disorder with depressed mood, and depressive disorder not otherwise specified.

The DSM-III-R definition of major depression corresponds almost exactly to that of DSM-III. A severity staging (mild, moderate, and severe), operationalized in a somewhat rudimentary way, is provided. The possibility of identifying a chronic subtype (when the current episodes lasts 2 consecutive years) is added.

The criteria for dysthymia require a 2-year period (not necessarily corresponding to the last 2 years) in which depressed mood was present for most of the day, with intervening periods of normal mood no longer than 2 months. Depressed mood must be accompanied by at least two of the six symptoms listed in Table 9.2, second column. There must be no major depressive episode in the first 2 years of the disorder (but these episodes may be superimposed later on), no previous manic or hypomanic episode, and no organic factor initiating and maintaining the disorder. It is possible to specify whether the disorder is primary or secondary and of early (before age 21) or late onset.

It is evident that the DSM-III-R concept of dysthymia has been narrowed with respect to that of DSM-III, following Akiskal's recommendations. The diagnosis should no longer be dysthymia if mild chronic depression develops as a sequela of a major depressive episode (in this case, the specifier "in partial remission" of major depression must be used) or is related to a medical condition; if it is linked to a preexisting psychiatric condition (other than a personality disorder), the secondary subtype of dysthymia must be applied. Moreover, following the suggestion of Kocsis and Frances (1987), the addition of an individual symptom is no longer sufficient to allow the shift from dysthymia to major depression. It is surprising, however, that, although Akiskal (1983) identified anhedonia as one of the main features of subaffective dysthymia, the "marked loss of interest or pleasure in usual activities," included in the DSM-III definition of dysthymic disorder, does not appear in DSM-III-R.

Hiller et al. (1988), in a study conducted on psychiatric outpatients in Germany, found that the DSM-III-R diagnoses most frequently corresponding to the ICD-9 category of neurotic depression were dysthymia and major depression (69% and 39% of cases, respectively, with the sum exceeding 100% because the two categories were sometimes used simultaneously). The discrepancy between these data and those reported in the above-mentioned studies (Perris et al., 1982; d'Elia et al., 1974) exploring the correspondence between ICD-9 neurotic depression and DSM-III dysthymic disorder may be taken as a further indication of the heterogeneous use of the former diagnostic label.

Winter et al. (1991) reported that 42% of patients received one of the not otherwise specified DSM-III-R diagnoses, and that in 70% of cases this was a diagnosis of depressive disorder not otherwise specified. As detailed above, 47% of these last cases fulfilled RDC for minor depression.

ICD-10

In ICD-10, published in 1992, "clinical descriptions and diagnostic guidelines" are given for the following depressive categories: depressive episode, recurrent depressive disorder, dysthymia, recurrent brief depressive disorder, brief and prolonged depressive reaction (included among adjustment disorders), and mixed anxiety and depressive disorder (included among "other anxiety disorders").

The severity staging for depressive episodes is more elaborate than that of DSM-III-R: Mild depressive episode is defined by the occurrence of two symptoms from a first list of three plus two symptoms from a second list of six, none of which should be intense; moderate depressive episode is characterized by the presence of two symptoms from the first list plus three or more from the second, some of which "are likely to be" intense; severe depressive episode is defined by the occurrence of all the symptoms from the first list plus at least four from the second, some of which must be intense. In spite of the imprecision (and of the uncertain reliability), this staging puts forward two concepts: (1) that the various depressive symptoms may have a different diagnostic "weight," and (2) that the severity of a depressive episode should be judged not only by the number of symptoms but also by their intensity.

The ICD-10 (World Health Organization, 1992) definition of dysthymia is not operationalized and does not contain elements of interest (incidentally, it incorporates the statement that "dysthymia has much in common with the concepts of depressive neurosis and neurotic depression" and lists these last concepts as inclusion terms). One notable difference from the DSM classification (which in principle permits frequent superposition of major depression of any severity on a preexisting dysthymia) is that ICD-10 superimposed episodes, if any, must not be severe.

The insertion of the categories of brief recurrent depressive disorder (defined by the occurrence about once a month during the past years of depressive episodes lasting less than 2 weeks but fulfilling symptomatic criteria for mild, moderate, or severe depressive episode) and mixed anxiety and depressive disorder (to be used when "symptoms of both anxiety and depression are present but neither, considered separately, is sufficiently severe to justify a diagnosis") reflects the preoccupation with a possible underdiagnosis of depressive disorders in general practice. In the previously cited general practice study by Winter et al. (1991), a mixed anxiety–depressive syndrome accounted for almost half of all the not otherwise specified DSM-III-R diagnoses, and 17% of the not otherwise specified depressive disorders lasted less than 2 weeks.

An important effect of the diffusion of ICD-10 is expected to be the increase of the comparability of U.S. epidemiological studies with European ICD-based case-register surveys, which report neurotic depression to be the most prevalent psychiatric diagnosis (Sytema et al., 1989).

DSM-IV

In DSM-IV (American Psychiatric Association, 1994), the definitions of major depression and dysthymia are nearly identical to the corresponding categories in DSM-III-R. It is notable that depressive neurosis is no longer parenthesized as a synonym for dysthymic disorders, whereas generalized loss of interest or pleasure is included. Curiously, the appendix of DSM-IV contains an "alternative" list of dysthymic criteria deriving from a field trial. These alternative criteria place greater emphasis on emotional–cognitive manifestations, whereas the definitive list in the body of DSM-IV tends to overrate classical vegetative symptoms. DSM-IV also recognizes the possibility that both major and dysthymic disorders might, in cross-section, present with reverse vegetative signs ("atypical features").

The residual category of depressive disorder not otherwise specified includes minor depressive disorder (a depressive syndrome lasting at least 2 weeks in which fewer of the five symptoms required for major depression are present) and recurrent brief depressive disorder (defined by depressive episodes lasting 2 days to 2 weeks, occurring at least once a month for 1 year). Moreover the residual category of anxiety disorder not otherwise specified includes a mixed anxiety–depressive disorder (in which clinically significant symptoms of anxiety and depression are present, but criteria for a specified anxiety or mood disorder are not met), and that of personality disorder not otherwise specified embodies, preceded by a question mark, a depressive personality disorder. For all the above disorders classified under residual categories, the Task Force on DSM-IV determined that the available information was insufficient to warrant acceptance in the official classification, but that systematic clinical research is to be encouraged.

Latest Attempts to Revive the Concept of Neurotic Depression

Among the latest proposals of revival of the concept of neurotic depression, those by Winokur's group (Winokur, 1985; Winokur et al., 1987; Tsuang & Winokur, 1992), Zimmerman et al. (1987), and Roth and Mountjoy (Chapter 8, this volume) must be mentioned.

Winokur (1985) submitted a set of criteria for neurotic–reactive depression, which require that the patient (1) meets Feighner's criteria (Klerman et al., 1979) for primary unipolar depression (almost identical to RDC for major depression); (2) has a stormy lifestyle (at least two of the following: divorce or separation; fired from job one or more times; quit job out of pique with no better one to replace it; multiple conflicts with coworkers, friends, family or in-laws; history of sexual problems); (3) attributes illness to a life event; (4) has at least three of the following symptoms: initial insomnia, self-pity, multiple somatic complaints, demanding behavior, hostility, depression reactive to circumstances; (5) either scores positively on a systematic personality test or fulfills one of the following: has shown lifelong irritability, continually abrogates responsibility, is hard to get along with, is chronic complainer about bodily functions, is easily upset, has major personality problems (inadequate personality); (6) has two or more nonserious suicide attempts; and (7) has no more than four among a miscellaneous list of items (including loss of interest in usual activities, retardation, delusions or hallucinations, self-condemnation, diurnal variation, early morning awakening and loss of concentration).

In support of this proposal, Winokur (1985) first reported that a family history of alcoholism was significantly more frequent in a sample of women with a clinical diagnosis of neurotic–reactive depression than in one with a diagnosis of endogenous depression, and that such a family history was significantly associated with some personality characteristics (demanding behavior, need for assurance, lifelong nervousness, complaining, and irritability). Subsequently, he carried out a study (Winokur et al., 1987) on a sample of patients meeting the DSM-III criteria for major depression, subdivided into a neurotic group (including those with a family history of alcoholism plus those whose depression was secondary to personality disorders, drug abuse, or neurotic disorders) and an endogenous group (including all other patients), and found that the former were younger at index, more likely to be divorced or separated, more likely to have had previous suicide attempts, and less likely to have shown marked improvement when treated with electroconvulsive therapy (ECT), and that their post-dexamethasone serum cortisol levels were significantly lower. Finally, Tsuang and Winokur (1992) applied the above-mentioned set of criteria for neurotic–reactive depression (with the exception of the one requiring a family history of alcoholism) in a sample of patients meeting DSM-III-R and Feighner's criteria for major depression and found that neurotic–reactive depressives, as compared with nonneurotic ones, had an earlier age at onset, a better outcome at discharge, a worse outcome at 3-year follow-up, a more frequent family history of alcoholism, a lower frequency of melancholia, and a higher likelihood to attribute their present illness to psychosocial stressors.

All the above three studies were retrospective and based on chart reviews. The second (Winokur et al., 1987) was seriously weakened by the criteria used for the subdivision of patients (neurotics were those who had either family history of alcoholism or a secondary depression; endogenous were all the others). In the third (Tsuang & Winokur, 1992), some of the features found to differentiate neurotics from nonneurotics were implicitly (e.g., absence of melancholia) or even explicitly (e.g., attribution of illness to a life event) embodied in the criteria initially used to diagnose neurotic–reactive depression.

Zimmerman et al. (1987) conceptualized neurotic depression as a unipolar major depression marked by six features: personality disturbance, psychosocial stress, age of onset before 40, blaming others for depression, nonserious suicide attempts, and history of marital separation or divorce. They tested this definition in a sample of patients fulfilling the DSM-III criteria for unipolar major depressive disorder. Patients with at least three of the above features were classified as neurotic, the others as nonneurotic. Neurotics were found to have a more frequent family history of alcoholism, a less frequent nonsuppression on the dexamethasone test, a lower likelihood to receive ECT, a lower improvement rate at discharge, and a higher readmission rate during a follow-up period of 6 months. Among the diagnostic criteria for neurotic depression proposed by Zimmerman et al. (1987), personality disturbance can in itself account for both some other diagnostic items (e.g., history of marital separation or divorce and psychosocial stress) and some validating features (e.g., family history of alcoholism or poor outcome), independently from the presence of depression, whereas age at onset before 40 is likely to have a poor reliability and specificity (in fact, it was found by Zimmerman et al., 1987, in 56% of patients classified as nonneurotic).

Roth and Mountjoy (Chapter 8, this volume) compiled, on the basis of a literature review, a list of the clinical characteristics of neurotic depression, including the following items: (1) symptoms—depressed mood lacking "distinct" quality, mood reactivity, somatic complaints with hypochondriacal concern, initial insomnia or interrupted sleep, no diurnal variation or worsening of symptoms in evening, prominent but variable anxiety, hostility or irritability, self-pity and tendency to blame others, absence of self-reproach or guilt, demanding and manipulative behavior, absence of psychomotor retardation; (2) personality—evidence of maladjustment, vulnerability in the premorbid personality that may color the symptomatology of illness; (3) life events—understandably related to onset of symptoms in a high proportion of cases; (4) course—usually episodic with clear remission; (5) family history—a history of affective disorders is usually lacking; and (6) treatment response—a proportion of patients respond to cognitive therapy, interpersonal psychotherapy, drugs, ECT, or a combination of these treatments. Of the foregoing items, the last three are clearly not specific enough to be used in an operational definition of neurotic depression, whereas that listed as (3) appears unsuitable to that purpose in light of the currently available evidence that neurotic and endogenous depression (identified on the basis of CATEGO) have the same likelihood to be preceded by a life stress (Bebbington et al., 1988); conversely, RDC situational depressions do not differ from nonsituational ones on any demographic, clinical, and psychosocial variable (Hirschfeld et al., 1985). One is left, therefore, with the usual association of the lack of melancholic features, the presence of the "self-pitying constellation" (Rosenthal & Gudeman, 1967), and the occurrence of personality disturbances, the ensemble of which 30 years of empirical research have been unable to validate as an independent clinical entity.

Conclusions

The first conclusion that can be drawn from the above survey is that there is no reason to revive the concept of neurotic depression. If this label merely connotes a nonendogenous depression with associated personality disturbances, one can simply use the nonmelancholic or nonendogenous subtype provided by currently available diagnostic systems, and search for one or more appropriate Axis II modifiers. These last should not necessarily be personality "disorders"; they may be personality "traits" or "features" (e.g., the presence of a certain number of items from the definition of histrionic personality disorder may be conceptualized as histrionic features and used as a modifier for the Axis I diagnosis of nonmelancholic depression). Different personality features may have different treatment implications (of course, not only as concerns the choice of drugs but also in regard to the selection of the most appropriate psychotherapeutic approach).

The second conclusion is that the reconceptualization of depressive temperament (Akiskal & Akiskal, 1992) is the most significant outcome of the research work centered on the DSM-III category of dysthymic disorder. The relationship between temperament and personality and whether a depressive temperament should appear on Axis II, or on Axis I as a subsyndromal affective illness, or on neither, are open issues.

In any case, it is plausible that a patient with a depressive temperament should not receive the same diagnosis as one with a nonendogenous depression complicated by histrionic personality features, and should not be treated in the same way.

Apart from the above, very important development, I do not believe that the current status of the concept of dysthymia is much better than that of neurotic depression. The time constraints that are part of the former concept, so arbitrary and difficult to apply reliably, appear to be redundant if applied to a depressive temperament, and probably inappropriate if adopted for nonendogenous depression with histrionic and/or dependent personality traits, whose course is usually capricious and unpredictable.

Finally, it would appear that the phenomenologically based RDC categories of depressive disorders are the most valid among the existing classifications, and the most suitable for use in different contexts, including general practice.

I suggest making them even more flexible, allowing both major and minor depressions to be subtyped as episodic or chronic, primary or secondary, and possibly melancholic or nonmelancholic. Moreover, I would provisionally delete the self-pitying constellation from the definition of minor depression, and I would stimulate a debate among psychiatrists about that pattern as a part of a more general reconsideration of the boundary between psychiatric symptoms and temperamental or personality features.

References

Akiskal, H. S. (1983). Dysthymic disorder: Psychopathology of proposed chronic depressive subtypes. *American Journal of Psychiatry, 14,* 11–20.

Akiskal, H. S., & Akiskal, K. F. (1992). Cyclothymic, hyperthymic, and depressive temperaments as subaffective variants of mood disorders. In A. Tasman &

M. B. Riba (Eds.), *Review of psychiatry* (Vol 11). Washington, DC: American Psychiatric Press.

Akiskal, H. S., Bitar, A. H., Puzantian, V. R., Rosenthal, T. L., & Walker, P. W. (1978). The nosological status of neurotic depression: A prospective three- to four-year follow-up examination in light of the primary–secondary and unipolar–bipolar dichotomies. *Archives of General Psychiatry, 35,* 756–766.

Akiskal, H. S., Rosenthal, T. L., Haykal, R. F., Lemmi, H., Rosenthal, R. H., & Scott-Strauss, A. (1980). Characterological depressions: Clinical and sleep EEG findings separating "subaffective dysthymias" from "character spectrum disorders." *Archives of General Psychiatry, 37,* 777–783.

American Psychiatric Association. (1968). *Diagnostic and statistical manual of mental disorders* (2nd ed.). Washington, DC: Author.

American Psychiatric Association. (1980). *Diagnostic and statistical manual of mental disorders* (3rd ed.). Washington, DC: Author.

American Psychiatric Association. (1987). *Diagnostic and statistical manual of mental disorders* (3rd ed., rev.). Washington, DC: Author.

American Psychiatric Association. (1994). *Diagnostic and statistical manual of mental disorders* (4th ed.). Washington, DC: Author.

Barrett, J. E., Barrett, J. A., Oxman, T. E., & Gerber, P. D. (1988). The prevalence of psychiatric disorders in a primary care practice. *Archives of General Psychiatry, 45,* 1100–1106.

Bebbington, P. E., Brugha, T., MacCarthy, B., Potter, J., Sturt, E., Wykes, T., Katz, R., & McGuffin, P. (1988). The Camberwell Collaborative Depression Study: I. Depressed probands: Adversity and the form of depression. *British Journal of Psychiatry, 152,* 754–765.

Carney, M. W. P., Roth, M., & Garside, R. F. (1965). The diagnosis of depressive syndromes and the prediction of ECT response. *British Journal of Psychiatry, 111,* 659–674.

d'Elia, G., von Knorring, L., & Perris, C. (1974). Non-psychotic depressive disorders: A ten year follow-up. *Acta Psychiatria Scandinavica, 50*(Suppl. 255), 173–186.

Feighner, J. P., Robins, E., Guze, S. B., Woodruff, R. A., Winokur, G., & Munoz, R. (1972). Diagnostic criteria for use in psychiatric research. *Archives of General Psychiatry, 26,* 57–63.

Hiller, W., Mombour, W., Rummler, R., & Mittelhammer, J. (1988). Divergence and convergence of diagnoses for depression between ICD-9 and DSM-III-R. *European Archives of Psychiatry and Neurological Sciences, 238,* 39–46.

Hirschfeld, R. M. A., Klerman, G. L., Andreasen, N. C., Clayton, P. J., & Keller, M. B. (1985). Situational major depressive disorder. *Archives of General Psychiatry, 42,* 1109–1114.

Kendell, R. E. (1976). The classification of depressions: A review of contemporary confusion. *British Journal of Psychiatry, 129,* 15–28.

Kielholz, P., Poldinger, W., & Adams, C. (1982). *Masked depression.* Koln-Lovenich: Deutscher Arzte-Verlag.

Kiloh, L. G., Andrews, G., Neilson, M., & Bianchi, G. N. (1972). The relationship of the syndromes called endogenous and neurotic depression. *British Journal of Psychiatry, 121,* 183–196.

Klerman, G. L., Endicott, J., Spitzer, R., & Hirschfeld, R. M. A. (1979). Neurotic depressions: A systematic analysis of multiple criteria and meanings. *American Journal of Psychiatry, 136,* 57–61.

Kocsis, J. H., & Frances, A. J. (1987). A critical discussion of DSM-III dysthymic disorder. *American Journal of Psychiatry, 144,* 1534–1542.

Paykel, E. S. (1986). American and European classifications of affective disorders. *Pharmacopsychiatry, 19,* 29–32.

Perris, C., Perris, H., Ericsson, U., & von Knorring, L. (1982). The genetics of depression: A family study of unipolar and neurotic–reactive depressed patients. *Archiv für Psychiatrie Nervenkrankheiten, 232,* 137–155.

Rosenthal, S. H., & Gudeman, J. E. (1967). The self-pitying constellation in depression. *British Journal of Psychiatry, 113,* 485–489.

Skodol, A. E., & Spitzer, R. L. (1983). ICD-9 and DSM-III: A comparison. In R. L. Spitzer, J. B. W. Williams, & A. E. Skodol (Eds.), *International perspectives on DSM-III.* Washington, DC: American Psychiatric Press.

Spitzer, R. L., Endicott, J., & Robin, E. (1975). *Research Diagnostic Criteria (RDC) for a selected group of functional disorders* (2nd ed.). New York: New York Psychiatric Institute, Biometrics Research Division.

Spitzer, R. L., & Wilson, P. T. (1975). Nosology and the official psychiatric nomenclature. In A. M. Freedman, H. I. Kaplan, & B. J. Sadock (Eds.), *Comprehensive textbook of psychiatry* (2nd ed., Vol. 1). Baltimore: Williams & Wilkins.

Sytema, S., Balestrieri, M., Giel, R., ten Horn, G. H. M. M., & Tansella, M. (1989). Use of mental health services in South Verona and Groningen. *Acta Psychiatria Scandinavica, 79,* 153–162.

Torgersen, S. (1986). Neurotic depression and DSM-III. *Acta Psychiatria Scandinavica, 73*(Suppl. 328), 31–34.

Tsuang, D. W., & Winokur, G. (1992). Testing the validity of the neurotic depression concept. *Journal of Nervous and Mental Disease, 180,* 446–450.

Wing, J. K., Cooper, J. E., & Sartorius, N. (1974). *Measurement and classification of psychiatric symptoms.* Cambridge, UK: Cambridge University Press.

Weissman, M. M., & Klerman, G. L. (1977). The chronic depressive in the community: Unrecognized and poorly treated. *Comprehensive Psychiatry, 18,* 523–532.

Winokur, G. (1985). The validity of neurotic–reactive depression: New data and reappraisal. *Archives of General Psychiatry, 42,* 1116–1122.

Winokur, G., Black, D. W., & Nasrallah, A. (1987). Neurotic depression: A diagnosis based on preexisting characteristics. *European Archives of Psychiatry and Neurological Science, 236,* 343–348.

Winter, P., Philipp, M., Buller, R., Delmo, C. D., Schwarze, H., & Benkert, O. (1991). Identification of minor affective disorders and implications for psychopharmacotherapy. *Journal of Affective Disorders, 22,* 125–133.

World Health Organization. (1974). *Glossary of mental disorders and guide to their classification, for use in conjunction with the International Classification of Diseases, 8th revision.* Geneva: Author.

World Health Organization. (1978). *Mental disorders: Glossary and guide to their classification in accordance with the ninth revision of the International Classification of Diseases.* Geneva: Author.

World Health Organization. (1992). *The ICD-10 classification of mental and behavioural disorders: Clinical descriptions and diagnostic guidelines.* Geneva: Author.

Zimmerman, M., Coryell, W., Stangl, D., & Pfohl, B. (1987). Validity of an operational definition for neurotic unipolar major depression. *Journal of Affective Disorders, 12,* 29–40.

CHAPTER 10

Beyond Neurasthenia and Chronic Fatigue

Donna B. Greenberg

This chapter explores the likelihood that some patients suffering from chronic fatigue states might have conditions distinct from anxiety and mood disorders. Both classes of disorders include fatigue as a major clinical manifestation. However, chronic fatigue syndrome (CFS), postviral fatigue syndrome (PVFS), and fibromyalgia evolved in the current medical and popular literature largely independent of the current concepts of depression and anxiety and the older literature on neurasthenia. Researchers sought a physical nonpsychiatric cause of chronic fatigue—a persistent virus, a neurological, rheumatological, or hormonal defect. Although major depressive disorder is common among these patients, the patients are heterogeneous and not all patients meet criteria for major depressive disorder at the time they are evaluated. The idea that chronic fatigue could be merely an equivalent of chronic depression has been anathema to patients and researchers. They seek a mechanism for persistent fatigue not yet revealed by consistent evidence of medical abnormality. However, teasing chronic fatigue, a symptom with an affective dimension, from dysphoria is not easy.

Fatigue and Effort

Fatigue has a complex relationship to effort, tension, and mood. William James (1908) offered a thoughtful description of these interrelationships in normal fatigue and in the medical problem of neurasthenia:

Everyone is familiar with the phenomenon of feeling more or less alive on different days. Every one knows on any given day that there are energies slumbering in him which the incitements of that day do not call forth, but which he might display if these were greater. Most of us feel as if a sort of cloud weighed upon us, keeping us below our highest notch of clearness in discernment, sureness in reasoning, or firmness in deciding. Compared with what we ought to be, we are only half awake. Our fires are damped, our drafts are checked. We are making use of only a small part of our possible mental and physical resources.

In some persons this sense of being cut off from their rightful resources is extreme, and we then get the formidable neurasthenic and psychasthenic conditions, with life grown into one tissue of impossibilities, that so many medical books describe. . . . The slightest functional exercise gives a distress which the patient yields to and stops. . . . A new range of power often comes in consequence of the bullying-treatment of efforts which the doctor obliges the patient, much against his will, to make. (pp. 14–16)

James compared the usual efficiency equilibrium to the nutritive equilibrium. Just as a man maintains a steady weight despite variable amounts of food intake, he maintains a steady level of energy at very different amounts of work once an equilibrium is set. This equilibrium is usually set well within a man's resources. Pushing beyond the first effective level of fatigue requires emotional excitements, unusual ideas of necessity, and efforts. These catalysts—excitement, necessity, and effort—are called into play sooner when energy is limited.

If the person is well, the movement is light, and no unpleasant consequences are expected, the task is effortless, James (1880) concluded in an earlier treatise. In patients who complain of fatigue on a chronic basis, volitional effort is required to move a muscle, to remember, to make a decision, and to attend to a disagreeable task. James's concept of volitional effort incorporated the will, ability to attend to the task, ability to tolerate disagreeable expectations, and resolution of conflict signified by consent to the discomfort. In depression, by its nature, all these components are impaired: Desire is low, attention disrupted, outlook pessimistic, and decisions difficult to resolve.

Those processes that normally require effort can be measured. Effortful cognitive processes include (1) tests of free recall, for instance, to recall a word on the tip of one's tongue, compared to word recognition; (2) delayed recall from short-term memory compared to working memory; and (3) memory of unrelated items compared to related ones. Perception of muscular effort is also measurable on the 15-point Borg scale which increases linearly with heart rate in young healthy adults (Borg, 1982; Lewis & Haller, 1991). These processes are impaired in major depressive disorder and Parkinson's disease and have been associated with dopaminergic dysfunction (Roy-Byrne et al., 1986; Weingartner et al., 1984; Cohen et al., 1982).

Tense Arousal and Affective Syndromes

Tense arousal colors the experience of energy and fatigue. In Thayer's (1989) model, energetic arousal or calm energy is associated with vigor and optimism. After the activity is completed, arousal declines and calm tiredness brings rest and inactivity. Sleep, relaxation, and recuperation occur in a state of low bodily resources and safety.

Thayer contrasts energetic (calm) arousal with tense arousal with anxiety or fear in the setting of real or imagined danger. Attention is focused on the threat. Muscles tense and preparations are made for emergency but not executed. If tension increases enough, the energy level begins to drop. As energy drops, the tone of tense arousal becomes more negative. Depression is associated with low energy but high tension.

Tense arousal and fatigue are features of all affective syndromes. Anxious neurotics were separated from depressives in part by the nature of the fatigue symptom. By definition, loss of zest and energy, the feeling of being slowed, was a criterion for depression; severe tension and inability to relax were features of anxiety (Roth et al., 1972). Anergic traits of easy fatigability, poor persistence, and marked reaction to minor physical complaints, such as heaviness in arms and legs, were seen as "characterological" features of somatization related to anxiety (Prusoff & Klerman, 1974). In patients with panic disorder, fatigue and the perception of below-normal physical endurance seem to be related to the severity of depressive symptoms (Greenberg et al., 1991). In hypomania, energetic arousal, focused attention, and action, may evolve to the frenetic, disorganized, dysphoric and anxious behavior associated with mania. The driven behavior, emotional lability, and tangential thinking become exhausting.

Fatigue States without Tension

However, not all fatigue is due to affective illness. There are conditions of fatigue not associated with tense arousal. Usually these have medical causes.

Patients have low-tension fatigue states after illness, surgery (Christensen et al., 1982), or radiation treatment (Greenberg et al., 1992) and usually recover. After viruses or other infections, subjective fatigue is associated with metabolic adjustments during this period of recovery. Often, for instance, triiodothyronine (T_3) decreases due to inhibition of the enzyme that converts thyroxine (T_4) to T_3. In some cases T_4 is low (Van Der Poll et al., 1990). The hypothalamus adjusts to the stress of illness. Pituitary production of thyroid stimulating hormone (TSH; thyrotropin) decreases (Wehmann et al., 1985), and nocturnal surges of TSH decrease as they do in hypothyroidism (Romijn & Wiersinga, 1990), but a normal response to thyrotropin releasing hormone (TRH) is preserved. As the patient recovers, TSH recovers first and may initially overshoot normal range. This low euthyroid state may be protein sparing (Wartofsky & Burman, 1982). Hypogonadal states of amenorrhea or low testosterone have been noted under stress. Usually, the organism returns to normal as recovery occurs.

Fatigue becomes chronic and physical endurance limited with neurological injury, cardiopulmonary disease, rheumatological disease, active cancer (Bruera & MacDonald, 1988), infection, hypothyroidism, Addison's disease, and myopathy. Specific drugs are associated with sedation, lethargy, or impairment of concentration: antihistamines, sedatives, narcotics, sympathetic antagonists, lithium, or occasionally serotonergic agonists.

Those treating patients complaining of chronic fatigue, with CFS, PVFS, or fibromyalgia have sought an organic etiology and treatment independent of anxiety and depression. The modern question about neurasthenic conditions is how fatigue and poor capacity for effort might persist in a low-tension, low-energy setting? Is it induced by an organic, "nonnervous" cause such as a virus? Are effortful or attentional processes specifically impaired by something besides depression? Is the commonly associated depressive state merely the result of secondary demoralization? Can neurasthenic conditions be distinguished from relapsing anxiety and depressive syndromes?

Chronic Fatigue Syndrome

In the mid-1980s, physicians hypothesized that certain cases of chronic fatigue were related to persistent viral infection. Epstein–Barr virus (EBV), the virus of mononucleosis, notorious for causing fatigue in adolescents, was the likely suspect. When the research focus turned away from EBV, the symptom cluster for chronic mononucleosis was clarified and renamed chronic fatigue syndrome. These criteria (Table 10.1) reflected a working case definition (Holmes et al., 1988). Most are subjective symptoms rather than signs; objective evidence of fever, pharyngitis, and lymphadenopathy has been found only infrequently. Most often physical signs are absent. The emphasis on upper respiratory infectious symptoms results from the original hypothesis of chronic mononucleosis and a high rate of atopy in the samples.

TABLE 10.1. Summary of the Working Case Definition of CFS

Both major criteria and either ≥ 6 symptomatic criteria plus ≥ 2 physical criteria or ≥ 8 symptomatic criteria must be present to fulfill the case definition.

Major criteria

1. Persistent or relapsing fatigue or easy fatigability that:
   a. Does not resolve with bed rest
   b. Is severe enough to reduce average daily activity by ≥ 50%
2. Other chronic clinical conditions have been satisfactorily excluded including preexisting psychiatric diseases

Minor criteria

Symptomatic or historical criteria: persistent or recurring symptoms lasting ≥ 6 months

1. Mild fever (37.5°C–38.6°C oral if documented by the patient) or chills
2. Sore throat
3. Lymph node pain in anterior or posterior cervical or axillary chain
4. Unexplained generalized muscle weakness
5. Muscle discomfort, myalgia
6. Prolonged (≥ 24 hours) generalized fatigue following previously tolerable levels of exercise
7. New, generalized headaches
8. Migratory noninflammatory arthralgia
9. Neuropsychological symptoms
   a. Photophobia
   b. Transient visual scotomata
   c. Forgetfulness
   d. Excessive irritability
   e. Confusion
   f. Difficulty thinking
   g. Inability to concentrate
   h. Depression
10. Sleep disturbance
11. Patient's description of initial onset of symptoms as acute or subacute

Physical criteria: documented by a physician on at least two occasions at least 1 month apart

1. Low-grade fever (37.6°C–38.6°C oral or 37.8°C–38.8°C rectal)
2. Nonexudative pharyngitis
3. Palpable or tender anterior or posterior cervical or axillary lymph nodes (< 2 cm in diameter)

Note. Adapted from Holmes et al. (1988). Copyright 1988 by The American College of Physicians. Adapted by permission.

Except for photophobia and transient visual scotomata, all the neuropsychiatric symptoms listed are commonly seen with depression. Patients with such major psychiatric diagnoses as bipolar disorder, psychotic depression, and substance abuse were excluded. The underlying assumption was that the cognitive and affective changes, headache, photophobia, and visual scotomata could represent a persistent viral encephalopathy. Although some groups have promoted the inclusion of criteria for immune deficiency because of reports of immune activation or various deficits, the committee on criteria did not think that the evidence for immune deficiency was consistent enough (Holmes, 1991; Herberman, 1991; Arnason, 1991). Formal studies of memory or concentration have not verified deficits in attention or effortful processes in those with CFS, although a subjective incapacity is reported (Grafman et al., 1991; Barofsky & Legron, 1991).

More recently, British research (Sharpe et al., 1991a) suggested that the definition of CFS includes patients whose fatigue has a definite time of onset, present at least 6 months and for more than 50% of the time. Fatigue must be severe and disabling and must affect both physical and mental functioning. Postinfection fatigue syndrome is a specified subtype lasting 6 months after an identified infectious illness.

Postviral Fatigue Syndrome

We live among viruses which at times cause acute systemic infection or encephalitis, but we have also become more knowledgeable about latent or persistent viruses that might damage the central nervous system. Acute viral malaise is usually associated with low energy, increased need for sleep rather than insomnia, and elevated cytokines. A latent virus such as herpes simplex I (HSV-I) might cause fatigue when reactivated as a fever blister. The fatigue dissipates as the ulcer heals. The rare HSV-I encephalitis is associated with fever, temporal lobe abnormalities, and antibodies in the spinal fluid. Fatigue is also a prominent symptom of active HIV, which causes direct damage to nerve cells and lethal immune suppression.

Although patients with CFS have been examined for evidence of viral infection, no one virus has been consistently implicated (Landay et al., 1991; Denman, 1990; Gold et al., 1990; Bell et al., 1988). Acute enterovirus infections often leave residua of myalgias and fatigue; titers of Coxsackie B have been evaluated and VP1, an associated antigen, measured. Yet the prevalence of specific viruses in patients with CFS has varied depending on the locale and how patients were selected (Levine et al., 1992). Serology to cytomegalovirus, EBV, HHV-6, and HIV have also been evaluated. One study showed increased gamma-interferon in the central spinal fluid of CFS patients, but serum levels of cytokines did not differ in two studies (Lloyd et al., 1991; Straus et al., 1989). However, no one virus and no one viral mechanism has been found.

Patients with CFS have a greater perception of muscular effort (Riley et al., 1990; Cohen et al., 1948; Rosen et al., 1990), but neuromuscular disorder has been excluded in these patients (Wessely & Powell, 1989;

Folgering & Snik, 1988; Lloyd et al., 1988; Stokes et al., 1988). The defect has been sought in the central nervous system rather than the muscle. Isolated reports of biochemical abnormalities, muscle fiber abnormalities, and mitochondrial damage under transmission electron microscopy would not explain central fatigue (Kennedy, 1991). Even the presence of persistent enterovirus RNA in muscle (Archard et al., 1988) does not clarify the mechanism of general disability over years.

One study of patients with myalgic encephalomyelitis found an isolated abnormality in the P_3 cognitive–event evoked-potential (Prasher et al., 1990). The finding means little without juxtaposed neuropsychiatric evaluation (Oken, 1990).

A mild central adrenal insufficiency due to subnormal corticotropin releasing hormone (CRH) or another central stimulus has also been suggested as an explanation for persistent fatigue in some patients with CFS (Demitrack et al., 1991). As in major depression, anorexia nervosa, and states of high cortisol, the adrenocorticotropin (ACTH) response to CRH stimulation was blunted. The adrenal was more sensitive to exogenous ACTH, but the maximal response was less. Demitrack and colleagues suggest that the adrenal cortex was hyperresponsive to ACTH as if ACTH exposure had previously been inadequate. These data are compatible with a deficiency of hypothalamic CRH or a deficiency of another arousal-producing neuropeptide. Because many of these patients had lifetime histories of affective illness, the possibility of blunted endocrine function between affective episodes is also a consideration. Glucocorticoid secretion may sometimes increase with remission of depression (Geracioti et al., 1992).

Fibromyalgia

Fibromyalgia, a syndrome of generalized muscular pain in which fatigue figured prominently, was once called neurasthenic musculoskeletal pain syndrome (Moldofsky & Scarisbrick, 1976). Because CFS included myalgias and arthralgias, the two syndromes overlap (Buchwald et al., 1987; Moldofsky et al., 1988). The significant physical signs of fibromyalgia are multiple points tender to palpation in muscle, at a bony prominence, or at muscle-bone interface (Wolfe et al., 1990). Sleep dysfunction, fatigue, and morning stiffness were seen commonly and were thought to be pathognomonic (Smythe & Moldofsky, 1977). Nonrestorative sleep, which was associated with specific electroencephalographic findings of persistent alpha waves during rapid eye movement (REM) and non-REM sleep, was thought important to the cause of the syndrome (Moldofsky & Lue, 1980).

New criteria developed by the American College of Rheumatology in 1990 redefined fibromyalgia as a condition of generalized pain and specific tender points (Table 10.2), eliminating fatigue. Fatigue occurred in 81%, sleep disturbance in 75%, and anxiety in 45–55% (Wolfe et al., 1990). Follow-up data show that most patients with fibromyalgia have recurrent pain (Felson, 1986), but prospective studies are yet to be done.

Two treatments have shown benefit in controlled studies: amitriptyline 25 mg, with and without naproxen (Carette et al., 1986; Goldenberg et al., 1986), and cyclobenzaprine (Bennett et al., 1988). These led to improvement in global physician assessment, in a measure of sleep quality and fatigue, and in tender point score. Mood was not assessed (Simms et al., 1991).

Differential Diagnosis

No specific laboratory abnormality or organic etiology has defined CFS, PVFS, and fibromyalgia. All three syndromes have been associated with

TABLE 10.2. The American College of Rheumatology 1990 Criteria for the Classification of Fibromyalgia

1. History of widespread pain

Definition: Pain is considered widespread when all of the following are present: pain in the left side of the body, pain in the right side of the body, pain above the waist, and pain below the waist. In addition, axial skeletal pain (cervical spine or anterior chest or thoracic spine or low back) must be present. In this definition, shoulder and buttock pain is considered as pain for each involved side. "Low back" pain is considered lower segment pain.

2. Pain in 11 of 18 tender point sites on digital palpitation

Definition: Pain, on digital palpation, must be present in at least 11 of the following 18 tender point sites:

Occiput: bilateral, at the suboccipital muscle insertions
Low cervical: bilateral, at the anterior aspects of the intertransverse spaces at C_5–C_7
Trapezius: bilateral, at the midpoint of the upper border
Supraspinatus: bilateral, at origins, above the scapula spine near the medial border.
Second rib: bilateral, at the second costochondral junctions, just lateral to the junctions on upper surfaces.
Lateral epicondyle: bilateral, 2 cm distal to the epicondyles.
Gluteal: bilateral, in upper outer quadrants of buttocks in anterior fold of muscle.
Knee: bilateral, at the medial fat pad proximal to the joint line.

Digital palpation should be performed with an approximate force of 4 kg.

For a tender point to be considered "positive,," the subject must state that the palpation was painful. "Tender" is not to be considered "painful."

Note. For classification purposes, patients will be said to have fibromyalgia if both criteria are satisfied. Widespread pain must have been present for at least 3 months. The presence of a second clinical disorder does not exclude the diagnosis of fibromyalgia. From Wolfe et al. (1990). Copyright 1990 by J. B. Lippincott. Reprinted by permission.

high rates of affective illness. Samples of patients with CFS have met criteria for psychiatric illness: major depressive disorder (35–75%), panic disorder (5%), dysthymia (5%), and somatization disorder (10–15%) (Abbey & Garfinkel, 1990). Fibromyalgia was associated with high rates of major depressive disorder (Hudson et al., 1985; Goldenberg, 1989) and irritable bowel syndrome (Yunus et al., 1989; Veale et al., 1991), another condition which some suggest should be included in the affective spectrum (Hudson & Pope, 1990; Hudson et al., 1992).

The patients who seek specialty care and ask for help may determine the definition of syndromes. Most studies of fibromyalgia reflect the patients referred to rheumatological specialists (Wolfe, 1990); most studies of CFS also reflect a referral population. Medical offices have acknowledged that fatigue and fatigability for which no medical diagnosis has been found are often due to anxiety and depression (Manu et al., 1989; Kroenke et al., 1988, Kirk et al., 1990).

CFS has been a diagnosis that people receive with anger, sometimes with the conviction of specific illness and an assumption that their suffering will be belittled as mental. Social and personality factors limit the acknowledgement of affective illness (Abbey & Garfinkel, 1991). Neurasthenia in China, which focuses on somatic rather than affective symptoms, was found to match the diagnosis of major depressive disorder by U.S. criteria (Kleinman, 1982). Somatization changes according to societal and medical definition (Shorter, 1992; Stewart, 1990).

CFS is heterogeneous. It is always difficult to know the nature of the subjects in a specific sample. The U.S. criteria are broad and vague, including fatigue after infection, relapsing affective disorder, allergic rhinitis, and fibromyalgia. No physical signs or laboratory data are pathognomonic. Major depressive disorder and chronic fatigue are often found together in part because the criteria themselves overlap. Katon and Russo (1992) have argued that the number of medically unexplained physical symptoms required to meet criteria for CFS inadvertently selects patients with the highest prevalence of lifetime psychiatric diagnoses, the tendency to amplify symptoms, and a greater degree of disability.

The criteria for CFS depend very much on patients' retrospective reports about fatigue and disability. In the case of PVFS, the patient attributes the problem to a previous febrile illness. Any who have cared prospectively for patients with affective illness know that patients often do not remember their level of function a few months past. They may not recognize the beginning of a depressive relapse and may attribute mood to the latest stressor, viral or otherwise. On the other hand, disappointment or anger at a given moment increases the intensity of symptoms, the cry of distress. Although criteria exclude substance abuse, bipolar illness, and eating disorder, sometimes by structured psychiatric interviews, an accurate history may be difficult to obtain. In clinical practice, history is augmented over multiple visits with medical records and sometimes reports of observers. These are diagnoses revealed over time in trusting relationships.

Some patients with a history of depressive illness but no acute episode may be in a poorly characterized phase of recuperation between episodes (Manu et al., 1989). We know that the spectrum of bipolar illness is multivariate; a manic patient may be elated, intoxicated, dysphoric, or phobic at different times (Klerman, 1981). Patients tend to go to the doctor when they do detect change, and the change from hypomania to depression may be particularly provocative because the patient sees the energy of hypomania as normal (Sharpe et al., 1991b). Others have suggested a common physiological abnormality accounting for comorbidity of fibromyalgia, irritable bowel syndrome, major depressive disorder, and panic disorder (Hudson et al., 1992) and the study of lifetime diagnoses and similar morbidity in families.

We need a better description of severe CFS when psychiatric syndromes are absent in order to define the contribution of fatigue alone. Otherwise, the phenomenon of depression will obscure the patients who may have a distinct organic deficit of low arousal without tension. The nature of the fatigue should be described by diurnal variation (Wood & Magnello, 1992), precipitating factors, duration, psychomotor signs, response to exercise, sedation, and attentional and effort defects. Specific neuropsychological tests to define deficits in attention and effort are necessary. Fatigue must be described in counterpoint to the longitudinal course of affective illness.

The first goal for patients with CFS is clarification of the symptom of fatigue (Barofsky & Legro, 1991) and the exclusion of medical causes. Depressive symptoms can be targeted for treatment with antidepressant medications. Psychodynamic issues for persistent symptoms vary. James's analysis of effort highlighted the components of motivation, necessity, tolerance for the disagreeable, and resolution of conflict. Some patients resist the "tyranny of the should"; others are angry that more effort would be required to accomplish their desires (Horney, 1950). Some have a compulsive need to work and only seek help long after overwork has brought incapacity (Rhoades, 1977). Others are perfectionistic, apt to tackle too much, fearful of success or failure, and easily frustrated (Burns, 1980).

CFS sometimes resembles somatoform pain disorder, with the spotlight on fatigue, depressive features, and the complications of increasing disability (Krupp et al., 1991; Blakely et al., 1991). Patients appear to have a low fatigue threshold, like a low pain threshold (Riley et al., 1990). They minimize emotional attributions (Powell et al., 1990). Treatments that focus

on necessity and optimum cognitive and aerobic function while acknow-
ledging the patient's suffering make common sense (Butler et al., 1991).
James (1908) would recognize these patients: some depressed and anxious;
others angry at being cut off from their rightful resources, and more angry
at the bullying treatment of doctors.

Conclusion

This chapter explores the difficulties of separating chronic fatigue and
related syndromes from anxiety, mood disorders, normal recovery, and the
fatigue of known medical disorders.

Fatigue has an affective dimension, a relation to effort, tension, and
mood. Tense fatigue is a feature of affective disorders. The modern
question about neurasthenic conditions—CFS, PVFS, and fibromyalgia—is
how fatigue might persist in a low-tension, low-arousal setting despite rest
without depression or anxiety. Recuperative states involving hypothalamic
adjustments are part of normal recovery. No specific virus or viral mechanism has been uncovered. Affective syndromes are prevalent in all three
syndromes. To find those few who may not have affective illness, the
symptom must be detailed and evaluated prospectively against the individual longitudinal course of affective illness. Until then, samples are heterogeneous, overlapping by definition, based on inadequate description and
retrospective evaluation of disability. Sensible treatment requires medical
evaluation, pharmacological treatment of affective symptoms, cognitive
and aerobic focus on necessary function, and appreciation of the patients'
suffering (Wessely & Sharpe, 1995).

The most recent criteria for the diagnosis of CFS (Fukada et al., 1994)
define a condition of severe mental and physical exhaustion—not somno-
lence or lack of motivation—a sensation that cannot be attributed to
exertion or diagnosed disease. They agree that chronic fatigue should be
able to be clinically evaluated, should not be otherwise explained, should
be persistent or relapsing with a new or definite onset, and should not be
due to ongoing exertion or substantially alleviated by rest. A key feature is
reduction in activities. Four or more of the following symptoms should
occur at the same time: self-reported impairment in short-term memory
or concentration severe enough to cause substantial reduction in activities;
sore throat; tender cervical or axillary lymph nodes, muscle pain, multijoint
pain without joint swelling or redness, headaches of a new type, pattern,
or severity; unrefreshing sleep; or postexertional malaise lasting more than
24 hours. Symptoms must have persisted or recurred during six or more
consecutive months and must not have predated fatigue.

Fukada and colleagues resolved the conflict about mood disorders by excluding the following conditions if they occurred within the previous 2 years: psychotic depression, bipolar disorder, schizophrenia, delusional disorder, anorexia nervosa, bulimia, and substance abuse (within 2 years before the onset of chronic fatigue or afterward). However, current anxiety, anxiety disorder, and nonmelancholic depression have not been excluded, so the challenge of teasing these conditions from the presentation of chronic fatigue remains.

References

Abbey, S. E., & Garfinkel, P. E. (1990). Chronic fatigue syndrome and the psychiatrist. *Canadian Journal of Psychiatry, 35,* 625–633.

Abbey, S. E., & Garfinkel, P. E. (1991). Neurasthenia and chronic fatigue syndrome: The role of culture in the making of a diagnosis. *American Journal of Psychiatry, 148,* 1638–1646.

Archard, L. E., Bowles, N. E., Behan, P. O., Bell, E. J., & Doyle, D. (1988). Postviral fatigue syndromes: Persistence of enterovirus RNA in muscle and elevated creatine kinase. *Journal of the Royal Society of Medicine, 81,* 326–329.

Arnason, B. G. W. (1991). Nervous system–immune system communication. *Reviews of Infectious Diseases, 13*(Suppl. 1), S134–S137.

Barofsky, I., & Legro, M. W. (1991). Definition and measurement of fatigue. *Reviews of Infection Diseases, 13*(Suppl. 1), S94–S97.

Bell, E. J., McCartney, R. A., & Riding, M. H. (1988). Coxsackie B viruses and myalgic encephalomyelitis. *Journal of the Royal Society of Medicine, 81,* 329–331.

Bennett, R. M., Gatter, R. A., Campbell, S. M., Andrews, R. P., Clark, S. R., & Scarola, J. A. (1988). A comparison of cyclobenzaprine and placebo in the management of fibrositis: A double-blind controlled study. *Arthritis and Rheumatism, 31,* 1535–1542.

Blakely, A. A., Howard, R. C., Sosich, R. M., Murdoch, J. C., Menkes, D. B., & Spears, G. F. (1991). Psychiatric symptoms, personality and ways of coping in chronic fatigue syndrome. *Psychological Medicine, 21,* 347–362.

Borg, G. A. V. (1982). Psychophysical bases of perceived exertion. *Medicine and Science in Sports and Exercise, 14,* 377–381.

Bruera, E., & MacDonald, R. N. (1988). Asthenia in patients with advanced cancer. *Journal of Pain Symptoms and Management, 3,* 9–14.

Buchwald, D., Goldenberg, D. L., Sullivan, J. L., & Komaroff, A. L. (1987). The "chronic active Epstein–Barr virus infection syndrome" and primary fibromyalgia. *Arthritis and Rheumatism, 30,* 1132–1136.

Burns, D. (1980). *Feeling good.* New York: Penguin.

Butler, S., Chalder, T., Ron, M., & Wessely, S. (1991). Cognitive behavior therapy in chronic fatigue syndrome. *Journal of Neurology, Neurosurgery and Psychiatry, 54,* 153–158.

Carette, S., McCain, G. A., Bell, D. A., & Fam, A. G. (1986). Evaluation of amitriptyline in primary fibrosisits. A double-blind, placebo-controlled study. *Arthritis and Rheumatism, 29,* 655–659.

Christensen, T., Bendix, T., & Kehlet, H. (1982). Fatigue and cardiorespiratory function following abdominal surgery. *British Journal of Surgery, 69,* 417–419.

Cohen, M. E., White, P. D., & Johnson, R. E. (1948). Neurocirculatory asthenia, anxiety neuroses or the effort syndrome. *Archives of Internal Medicine, 81,* 260–281.

Cohen, R. M., Weingartner, H., Smallberg, S. A., Pickar, D., & Murphy, D. L. (1982). Effort and cognition in depression. *Archives of General Psychiatry, 39,* 593–598.

Demitrack, M. A., Dale, J. K., Straus, S. E., Laue, L., Listwak, S. J., Kruesi, J. J., Chrousos, G. P., & Gold, P. W. (1991). Evidence for impaired activation of the hypothalamic-pituitaryadrenal axis in patients with chronic fatigue syndrome. *Journal of Clinical Endocrinology and Metabolism, 73,* 1224–1234.

Denman, A. M. (1990). The chronic fatigue syndrome: A return to common sense. *Postgraduate Medical Journal, 66,* 499–451.

Folgering, H., & Snik, A. (1988). Hyperventilation syndrome and muscle fatigue. *Journal of Psychosomatic Research, 32,* 165–171.

Fukada, K., Straus, S., Hickie, I., Sharpe, M. C., Dobbins, J. G., & Komaroff, A. (1994). The chronic fatigue syndrome: A comprehensive approach to its definition and study. *Annals of Internal Medicine, 121,* 953–959.

Geracioti, T. D., Loosen, P. T., Gold, P. W., & Kling, M. A. (1992). Cortisol, thyroid hormone, and mood in atypical depression: A longitudinal case study. *Biological Psychiatry, 31,* 515–519.

Gold, D., Bowden, R., Sixbey, J., Riggs, R., Katon, W. J., Ashley, R., Obrigewitch, R. M., & Corey, L. (1990). Chronic fatigue, a prospective clinical and virologic study. *Journal of the American Medical Association, 264,* 48–53.

Goldenberg, D. L. (1989). Psychiatric and psychologic aspects of fibromyalgia syndrome. *Rheumatic Disease Clinics of North America, 15,* 105–114.

Goldenberg, D. L., Felson, D. T., & Dinerman, H. (1986). A randomized, controlled trial of amitriptyline and naproxen in the treatment of patients with fibromyalgia. *Arthritis and Rheumatism, 29,* 1371–1377.

Grafman, J., Johnson, R., & Scheffers, M. (1991). Cognitive and mood-state changes in patients with chronic fatigue syndrome. *Reviews of Infectious Diseases, 13*(Suppl 1), S45–52.

Greenberg, D. B., Eisenthal, S., Tesar, G. E., Rosenbaum, J., Pollack, M. H., Herman, J. B., Sachs, G., & Cohen, L. S. (1991). Linking panic disorder and depression: The fatigue dimension. *Annals of Clinical Psychiatry, 3,* 205–208.

Greenberg, D. B., Sawicka, J., Eisenthal, S., & Ross, D. (1992). Fatigue syndrome due to localized radiation. *Journal of Pain and Symptom Management, 7,* 38–45.

Herberman, R. B. (1991). Sources of confounding in immunologic data. *Reviews of Infectious Diseases, 13*(Suppl. 1), S84–S86.

Holmes, G. P. (1991). Defining the chronic fatigue syndrome. *Reviews of Infectious Diseases, 13*(Suppl. 1), S53–S55.

Holmes, G. P., Kaplan, J. E., Gantz, N. M., Komaroff, A. L., Schonberger, L. B., Straus, S. E., Jones, J. F., Dubois, R. E., Cunningham-Rundles, C., Pahwa, S., et al. (1988). Chronic fatigue syndrome: A working case definition. *Annals of Internal Medicine, 108,* 387–389.

Horney, K. (1950). *Neurosis and human growth.* New York: W. W. Norton.

Hudson, J. I., Goldenberg, D. L., Pope, H. G., Keck, P. E., Jr., & Schlesinger, L. (1992). Comorbidity of fibromyalgia with medical and psychiatric disorders. *American Journal of Medicine, 92,* 363–367.

Hudson, J. I., Hudson, M. S., & Pliner, L. F., Goldenberg, D. L., & Pope, H. G., Jr. (1985). Fibromyalgia and major affective disorders. A controlled phenomenology and family history study. *American Journal of Psychiatry, 142,* 441–446.

Hudson, J. I., & Pope, H. G. (1990). Affective spectrum disorder: Does antidepressant response identify a family of disorders with a common pathophysiology? *American Journal of Psychiatry, 147,* 552–564.

James, W. (1880). The feeling of effort. In *Anniversary memoirs of the Boston Society of Natural History* (pp. 3–32). Boston: Boston Society of Natural History.

James, W. (1908). The energies of men . In *Religion and medicine* (pp. 12–16). New York: Moffat, Yard & Co.

Katon, W., & Russo, J. S. (1992). Chronic fatigue syndrome criteria. *Archives of Internal Medicine, 152,* 1604–1609.

Kennedy, P. (1991). Postviral fatigue syndrome current neurobiological perspective. *British Medical Bulletin, 47,* 809–814.

Kirk, J., Douglass, R., Nelson, E., Jaffe, J., Lopez, A., Ohler, J., Blanchard, C., Chapman, R., McHugo, G., & Stone, K. (1990). Chief complaint of fatigue: A prospective study. *Journal of Family Practice, 30,* 33–41.

Kleinman, A. (1982). Neurasthenia and depression. A study of somatization and culture in China. *Culture, Medicine, and Psychiatry, 6,* 117–190.

Klerman, G. L. (1981). The spectrum of mania. *Comprehensive Psychiatry, 22,* 11–19.

Kroenke, K., Wood, D. R., Mangelsforff, A. D., Meier, N. J., & Powell, J. B. (1988). Chronic fatigue in primary care. *Journal of the American Medical Association, 260,* 929–934.

Krupp, L. B., Mendelson, W. B., & Friedman, R. (1991). An overview of chronic fatigue syndrome. *Journal of Clinical Psychiatry, 52,* 403–410.

Landay, A. L., Jessop, C., Lennette, E. T., & Levy, J. A. (1991). Chronic fatigue syndrome: Clinical condition associated with immune activation. *Lancet, 338,* 707–712.

Levine, P. H., Jacobson, S., Pocinki, A. G., Cheney, P., Peterson, D., Connelly, R. R., Weil, R., Robinson, S. M., Ablashi, D. V., Salahudoin, S. Z., et al. (1992). Clinical, epidemiologic, and virologic studies in four clusters of the chronic fatigue syndrome. *Archives of Internal Medicine, 152,* 1611–1616.

Lewis, S. F., & Haller, R. G. (1991). Physiologic measurement of exercise and fatigue with special reference to chronic fatigue syndrome. *Reviews of Infectious Diseases, 13*(Suppl. 1), S98–S108.

Lloyd, A. R., Hales, J. P., & Gandevia, S. C. (1988). Muscle strength, endurance and recovery in the post-infection fatigue syndrome. *Journal of Neurology, Neurosurgery, and Psychiatry, 51,* 1316–1322.

Lloyd, A., Hickie, I., Brockman, A., Dwyer, J., & Wakefield, D. (1991). Cytokine levels in serum and cerebrospinal fluid in patients with chronic fatigue syndrome and control subjects. *Journal Infectious Diseases, 164,* 1023–1024.

Manu, P., Matthews, D. A., Lane, T. J., Tennen, H., Hesselbrock, V., Mendola, R., & Affleck, G. (1989). Depression among patients with a chief complaint of chronic fatigue. *Journal of Affective Disorders, 17,* 165–172.

Moldofsky, H., & Lue, F. A. (1980). The relationship of alpha and delta EEG frequencies to pain and mood in "fibrositis" patients treated with chlorpromazine and l-tryptophan. *Electroencephalography and Clinical Neurophysiology, 50,* 71–80.

Moldofsky, H., Saskin, P., & Lue, F. A. (1988). Sleep and symptoms in fibrositis syndrome after a febrile illness. *Journal of Rheumatology, 15,* 1701–1704.

Moldofsky, H., & Scarisbrick, P. (1976). Induction of neurasthenic musculoskeletal pain syndrome by selective sleep state deprivation. *Psychosomatic Medicine, 38,* 35–44.

Oken, B. S. (1990). Endogenous event-related potentials. In K. H. Chiappa (Ed.), *Evoked potentials in clinical medicine* (2nd ed., pp. 563–578). New York: Raven Press.

Powell, R., Dolan, R., & Wessely, S. (1990). Attributions and selfesteem in depression and chronic fatigue syndromes. *Journal of Psychosomatic Research, 34,* 665–673.

Prasher, D., Smith, A., & Findley, L. (1990). Sensory and cognitive event-related potentials in myalgic encephalomyelitis. *Journal of Neurology, Neurosurgery, and Psychiatry, 53,* 247–253.

Prusoff, B., & Klerman, G. L. (1974). Differentiating depressed from anxious neurotic outpatients. *Archives of General Psychiatry, 30,* 302–309.

Rhoades, J. M. (1977). Overwork. *Journal of the American Medical Association, 237,* 2615–2618.

Riley, M. S., O'Brien, C. J., McCluskey, D. R., Bell, N. P., & Nicholls, D. P. (1990). Aerobic work capacity in patients with chronic fatigue syndrome. *British Medical Journal, 301,* 953–956.

Romijin, J. A., & Wiersinga, W. M. (1990). Decreased nocturnal surge of thyrotropin in nonthyroidal illness. *Journal of Clinical Endocrinology and Metabolism, 70,* 35–42.

Rosen, S. D., King, J. C., Wilkinson, J. B., & Nixon, P. G. F. (1990). Is chronic fatigue syndrome synonymous with effort syndrome? *Journal of the Royal Society of Medicine, 83,* 761–764.

Roth, M., Gurney, C., Garside, R. F., & Kerr, T. A. (1972). Studies in the classification of affective disorder. The relationship between anxiety states and depressive illness: I. *British Journal of Psychiatry, 121,* 147–161.

Roy-Byrne, P. P., Weingartner, H., Bierer, L. M., Thompson, K., & Post, R. M. (1986). Effortful and automatic cognitive processes in depression. *Archives of General Psychiatry, 43,* 265–267.

Sharpe, M. C., Archard, L. C., Banatvala, J. E., Borysiewicz, L. K., Clare, A. W., David, A., Edwards, R. H., Hawton, K. E., Lambert, H. P., Lane, R. J., et al. (1991a). A report of chronic fatigue syndrome: Guidelines for research. *Journal of the Royal Society of Medicine, 84,* 118–121.

Sharpe, M. C., Johnson, B. A., & McCann, J. (1991b). Mania and recovery from chronic fatigue syndrome. *Journal of the Royal Society of Medicine, 84,* 51–54.

Shorter, E. (1992). *From paralysis to fatigue: A history of psychosomatic illness in the modern era.* Toronto: Free Press.

Simms, R. W., Felson, D. T., & Goldenberg, D. L. (1991). Development of preliminary criteria for response to treatment in fibromyalgia syndrome. *Journal of Rheumatology, 18,* 1558–1563.

Smythe, H. A., & Moldofsky, H. (1977). Two contributions to understanding of the "fibrositis" syndrome. *Bulletin of Rheumatic Disease, 28,* 928–931.

Stewart, D. E. (1990). The changing faces of somatization. *Psychosomatics, 31,* 153–158.

Stokes, M. J., Cooper, R. G., & Edwards, R. H. T. (1988). Normal muscle strength and fatiguability in patients with effort syndromes. *British Medical Journal, 297,* 1014–1017.

Straus, S. E., Dale, J. K., Peter, J. B., & Dinarello, C. A. (1989). Circulating lymphokine levels in the chronic fatigue syndrome. *Journal of Infectious Diseases, 160,* 1085–1086.

Thayer, R. E. (1989). *The biopsychology of mood and arousal.* New York: Oxford University Press.

van der Poll, T., Romijn, J. A., Wiersinga, W. M., & Sauerwein, H. P. (1990). Tumor necrosis factor: A putative mediator of the sick euthyroid syndrome in man. *Journal of Clinical Endocrinology and Metabolism, 71,* 1567–1572.

Veale, D., Kavanagh, G., Fielding, J. F., & Fitzgerald, O. (1991). Primary fibromyalgia and the irritable bowel syndrome: Different expressions of a common pathogenetic process. *British Journal of Rheumatology, 30,* 220–222.

Wartofsky, L., & Burman, K. D. (1982). Alterations in thyroid function in patients with systemic illness: The "euthyroid sick syndrome." *Endocrine Reviews, 3,* 164–217.

Wehmann, R. E., Gregerman, R. I., & Burns, W. H., Saral, R., & Santos, G. W. (1985). Suppression of thyrotropin in the low-thyroxine state of severe nonthyroidal illness. *New England Journal of Medicine, 312,* 546–552.

Weingartner, H., Burns, S., Diebel, R., & Lewitt, P. A. (1984). Cognitive impairments in Parkinson's disease: Distinguishing between effortful and automatic cognitive processes. *Psychiatry Research, 11,* 223–225.

Wessely, S., & Powell, R. (1989). Fatigue syndromes: A comparison of chronic "postviral" fatigue with neuromuscular and affective disorders. *Journal of Neurology, Neurosurgery and Psychiatry, 52,* 940–948.

Wessely, S., & Sharpe, M. (1995). Chronic fatigue, chronic fatigue syndrome, and fibromyalgia. In R. Mayou, C. Bass, & M. Sharpe (Eds.), *Treatment of functional somatic symptoms* (pp. 285–312). New York: Oxford University Press.

Wolfe, F. (1990). Fibromyalgia. *Rheumatic Disease Clinics of North America, 16,* 681–698.

Wolfe, F., Smythe, H. A., Yunus, M. B., Bennett, R.M., Bombardier, C., Goldenberg, D. L., Tugwell, P., Campbell, S. M., Abeles, M., Clark, P., et al. (1990). The American College of Rheumatology 1990 criteria for classification of fibromyalgia: Report of the multicenter criteria committee. *Arthritis and Rheumatism, 33,* 160–172.

Wood, C., & Magnello, M. E. (1992). Diurnal changes in perceptions of energy and mood. *Journal of the Royal Society of Medicine, 85,* 191–194.

Yunus, M. B., Masi, A. T., & Aldag, J. C. (1989). A controlled study of primary fibromyalgia syndrome: Clinical features and association with other functional syndromes. *Journal of Rheumatology, 16*(Suppl. 19), 62–71.

CHAPTER 11

Atypical Depressions

Jonathan R. T. Davidson

The concept of atypical depression as a specifically monoamine oxidase inhibitor (MAOI)-responsive disorder arose more than 30 years ago. It has continued to fascinate psychiatrists, yet there is no consensus on the core characteristics of this affective subtype. With the arrival of new non-MAOI antidepressants, it is likely that atypical depression will be found to respond well to these compounds as well. This chapter examines five different renditions of the term "atypical" as they relate to MAOI effects; it also assesses issues of construct validity and the contributions made by multivariate grade of membership studies to the establishment of atypical depression as a nosological entity.

Historical and Terminological Aspects

In 1959, West and Dally reported salutary effects of iproniazid, an MAOI, in depressed patients who did not exhibit classical symptoms of endogenous depression. Because, at that time, endogenous depression was considered to be the typical form of depression, the MAOI-responsive state was termed "atypical depression." Others (Sargant & Dally, 1962; Pollitt, 1965; Lascelles, 1965) used the same term to describe an even broader spectrum of affective patients who appeared to show a favorable response to MAOIs. They included syndromes that showed conspicuously prominent phobic anxiety, autonomic arousal, reversal of the usual vegetative symptoms, irritability and so-called hysterical features, and, finally, chronic pain.

During the past three decades, the rubric of "atypical depression" has been widely used, but regrettably without any serious attempt to establish whether it comprised nonoverlapping subtypes or was, in fact, a discrete entity. Yet there are at least five meanings of the term that we recognize today (Davidson et al., 1982):

1. Nonendogenous depression
2. Depression with reversal of vegetative symptoms
3. Depression with prominent panic or phobic symptoms
4. Depression with rejection or interpersonal sensitivity
5. Depression with chronic pain

This chapter examines the importance of each definition vis-à-vis response to MAOI and other antidepressant therapy. It also examines whether different usages of the term overlap, as would be expected if atypical depression were a unitary construct. Finally, this chapter revisits atypical depression as a type of depression that receives support from multivariate classification studies.

Relation between the Various Definitions and MAOI Response

Nonendogenous Depression

Is the endogenous versus nonendogenous dichotomy meaningful with respect to MAOI treatment? There is now little doubt that MAOIs are effective in endogenous depression (Davidson et al., 1987, 1988a; Nolen, 1986; Kiloh et al., 1959). Although in more severe forms of depression their efficacy may be diminished (Davidson et al., 1986, 1987) it adds little to say that nonendogenous depression is atypical and/or that it is essentially MAOI responsive.

However, two interesting leads have emerged from studies with isocarboxazid, which serve to validate the construct of nonendogenicity without necessarily supporting the case of atypicality. Thus, we found a positive correlation between antidepressant effects and platelet monoamine oxidase inhibition in Research Diagnostic Criteria (RDC)-defined nonendogenous depression, but not in endogenous depression (Davidson et al., 1986).

In a second study (Davidson & Turnbull, 1984), we demonstrated that a high dose of isocarboxazid was more effective than a low dose in nonendogenous depression, but that a comparable dose–response relationship did not pertain to endogenous depression.

Reversed Vegetative Symptoms

In the most widely used definition of atypicality, established by the Columbia group (Liebowitz et al., 1984), increased appetite, weight gain, and hypersomnia are part of the diagnostic criteria. Widely believed to be important to the concept, there is no firm evidence yet that their presence is essential to, or accounts for, the specific effects of MAOIs. Two of my studies have, in fact, found this not to be the case (Davidson & Pelton, 1986; Davidson et al., 1988a).

The reversed vegetative symptom of increased libido, although distinctly less common, may be more closely connected to certain forms of "hysteroid depression," and was described by Sargant and Slater (1972) as predicting good response to an MAOI. Stability of reversed vegetative symptoms across episodes has been shown by Nierenberg et al. (1996).

Panic and Phobic Symptoms

In analyzing pooled data from a variety of MAOI trials conducted in our center, the presence of panic symptoms was found to be associated with greater response to MAOIs than to tricyclic antidepressants (TCAs) in women, although the reverse was true for men (Davidson & Pelton, 1986).

In a study by Robinson et al. (1985), depression with panic attacks was associated with preferential response to phenelzine relative to imipramine. Another report from our center (Davidson et al., 1987) found a similar difference in favor of phenelzine over imipramine. Finally, Liebowitz et al. (1984) also found a difference in favor of phenelzine over imipramine in atypical depression with panic attacks.

Only one study has examined the relative contribution made by panic attacks and phobic symptoms to MAOI effects while controlling for the possible effects of other atypical features. In our multicenter report of isocarboxazid and placebo in atypical depression (Davidson et al., 1988a), we noted that the influence of panic attacks was outweighed by the influence of phobic avoidance and interpersonal sensitivity.

Interpersonal Sensitivity

Clinical observations made by West and Dally (1959) and Klein et al. (1985) suggested that interpersonal or rejection hypersensitivity was an important predictor of MAOI response and TCA nonresponse. This was first demonstrated prospectively by the Columbia group (Liebowitz et al., 1984); in this study, evaluating phenelzine and imipramine versus placebo, rejection sensitivity was actually included as one of the diagnostic criteria for atypical depression.

In the Duke study of isocarboxazid and placebo (Davidson et al., 1988a), we found interpersonal sensitivity (IPS) to be the most significant predictor of MAOI effects. Its contribution, in a linear regression model, outweighed the contributions of five other atypical features: panic, phobia, vegetative reversal, hostility, and somatic anxiety. However, it is noteworthy that the overall variance explained by these atypical features was low, indicating that other variables could be as important. Such variables as being female, absence of concomitant medical disorder, absence of prior psychiatric hospitalization, presence of precipitating factors, and nonreactivity of mood were all found to be predictive of outcome in a separate analysis of our sample (Davidson et al., 1991).

An important difference between the Duke and the Columbia studies rests in their somewhat different operationalization of IPS. The former definition is based on a clinical evaluation of rejection sensitivity as a personality style (an exaggerated version of which has been referred to as "hysteroid dysphoria" [Klein et al., 1985]), whereas the Duke study used a measure of IPS taken from the Hopkins Symptom Checklist–58 (Derogatis et al., 1974). The relationship between these two IPS constructs is unclear.

In another study of IPS (Davidson et al., 1989a), we made several observations that suggest that the study of IPS merits more intensive study.

As defined by us, IPS consisted of six items: feeling critical of others, feeling being easily hurt, feeling that others are neither understanding nor sympathetic, feeling others are unfriendly, feeling inferior to others, and feeling shy or uneasy with the opposite sex. Those with high IPS symptoms were distinguishable from those with lower IPS by being more depressed, having more frequent familial schizophrenia, earlier onset of depression, and more chronic depression. Thus, depression lasted an average of 39 months in high IPS patients, compared to 19–26 months in lower IPS groups.

Symptomatologically, high IPS depression was more commonly associated with overeating or weight gain, panic attacks, and phobic symptoms. IPS was found to be unrelated to the concept of endogenicity (i.e., one was not a manifestation of the other) and overlap was not present. High IPS depression was also related to higher severity of "peripheral" symptoms (e.g., self-referential thinking and depersonalization or derealization).

An interesting relationship emerged between baseline IPS score and treatment response to isocarboxazid and placebo. Placebo effects diminished and medication effects increased as the baseline IPS score increased. At low levels of IPS, there was no difference in outcome using the final score the Hamilton Rating Scale for Depression (Hamilton, 1960) a difference of 0.2 was observed between active medication and placebo. In the midrange IPS group, the difference was 9.8, and in the high IPS group the difference was 12.2.

The construct of interpersonal sensitivity deserves further in-depth study. It would be important to develop a reliable observer rating and also to compare the relative importance of IPS as symptoms and as a personality trait to the issues addressed here. Some strides have been made in this direction by Boyce et al. (1991), who developed a questionnaire to measure IPS as a predictor of subsequent depression. Actually, IPS may underlie atypicality in anxious–phobic and bipolar II depressives (Akiskal et al., 1995).

With the advent of a new generation of antidepressants—such as bupropion and the selective serotonin reuptake inhibitors (SSRIs), as well as the selective, reversible MAOIs—the foregoing issues need to be brought to bear on the therapeutic effects of these new agents. Their utility in treating atypical depression needs to be evaluated, particularly in view of the untoward risk and side effects of the older MAOIs. Two more recent studies using the Columbia definition of atypical depression have found gepirone, a 5-HT_{1A} partial agonist, to be superior to placebo (McGrath et al., 1994), as well as a high response rate for fluoxetine and phenelzine (Pande et al., 1996).

Chronic Pain

An early study by Lascelles (1956) showed greater therapeutic efficacy for phenelzine over placebo in atypical facial pain, and a later study by Raft et al. (1979) showed greater improvement from phenelzine, as compared to amitriptyline and placebo, in a population of major depressives with chronic pain.

An interesting relationship thus exists between chronic pain, atypicality and MAOI response. In the Raft et al. (1979) study, the great majority of patients exhibited atypical vegetative symptoms and rejection sensitivity (Davidson & Raft, 1985). Another study (Davidson et al., 1985) by our group on chronic low back pain also revealed a high rate of reverse vegetative signs. Further studies in this patient population would be likely to shed more light in defining the phenomenology of atypical depressions.

Overlapping or Distinct Constructs?

There has been little work as to the degree of overlap, but two studies suggest the overlap is minimal. We have found that endogenous depression and IPS did not bear a meaningful relationship to each other: Numbers of endogenous and nonendogenous depressives did not differ according to IPS status on three of four measures of endogenicity (Davidson et al., 1989a).

Paykel et al. (1983) found minimal overlap between three definitions of atypicality: Newcastle nonendogenous, ICD-10 neurotic, and vegetative reversal. The authors concluded that atypical depression may be of limited value as a specific diagnosis within nonpsychotic depression. However, the basis for this conclusion rests on the use of only three definitions of atypicality. It is noteworthy, nonetheless, that these authors did report that no matter how defined, atypicality did not preclude response to the TCA amitriptyline.

Early multivariate studies of depression nosology repeatedly isolated endogenous and nonendogenous depressions but said little about the existence of atypical depression. This is not surprising because these studies did not include the relevant symptoms (i.e., panic attacks, phobias, vegetative reversal, and IPS).

Two recent reports using grade of membership (GOM) analysis have proved illuminating and do provide some validation of the notion(s) of atypical depression. GOM is a relatively new technique, developed for the purposes of classifying medical disease or symptoms. It permits simultaneous assignment of symptoms (or phenomena) into groups and people into disease type. It operates on the "fuzzy set" principle, which assumes that most people (patients) belong particularly to more than one group, although it is possible to assign a person to one group on the basis of predominant group membership. The background and applications of GOM have been described elsewhere (Davidson et al., 1988c). In this chapter I summarize two of my studies that provide some support of the concept of atypical depression.

In the first study (Davidson et al., 1988c), five pure types of depression were isolated from a pool of patients that included typical and atypical patients. All cases of hyperphagia clustered into one pure (atypical) type, and all severe cases of panic attacks clustered into two (atypical) pure types. Thus, several types did resemble atypical depression, although only a minority (approximately 20%) exhibited vegetative reversal even in the group that showed the highest clustering of atypical symptoms.

The second GOM study (Davidson et al., 1989b) also isolated five depressive types, one of which exhibited more clearly than the other types most of the atypical features we have reviewed (Davidson et al., 1988a). IPS, panic attacks, and vegetative reversal were especially common in this pure type. It was accompanied by evidence of "character" pathology and showed greater response to an MAOI than to placebo. It must be said, however, that response rates overall were low in this type.

These two multivariate studies of depressive nosology do provide some support for the construct of atypical depression; the interrelations between the various components of atypicality still await clarification.

It is finally noteworthy that hypersomnic–hyperphagic dysthymics with classical diurnality (i.e., morning worsening of mood) have been described by Akiskal et al. (1980). These patients often meet the criteria of a depressive personality type yet seem to respond to desipramine-type agents with hypomania. These patients might also belong to a special atypical depressive subgroup (Davidson et al., 1982).

Conclusion

The concept of atypical depression continues to fascinate psychiatrists. The principal reason for this fascination lies in an enduring belief, dating back to the 1950s when MAOIs and TCAs were the only pharmacological choices for depression, that MAOIs have a preferential effect relative to TCA and placebo in this subtype. Studies to date have generally upheld this belief.

However, the relevance of the question may have diminished, now that many alternative groups of antidepressants are becoming available, such as the aminoketone, SSRIs, and azapirones. It is widely believed that these agents can be as effective as MAOIs in atypical depression, but direct comparisons have not yet been published. A number of clinical trials are now under way to establish their effects in atypical depression.

As an overall summary of the existing literature, it would be fair to say that atypical depression does not respond well to the two traditional TCAs (imipramine and amitriptyline), although atypical depression is TCA responsive, but that MAOIs are equally effective in atypical and typical depression.

To date, there have been few validating studies to support the existence of a true atypical depressive subtype, and there is no universally agreed consensus for any particular core characterization of the disorder. At this time, it appears as though IPS may be the most fruitful area to study in this regard. High levels of IPS in turn may be more likely to carry an association with reverse vegetative symptomatology and possibly panic or phobia. This might eventually explain the link between several definitional characteristics of atypical depressions.

References

Akiskal, H. S., Maser, J. D., Zeller, P. J., Endicott, J., Coryell, W., Keller, M., Warshaw, M., Clayton, P., & Goodwin, F. (1995). Switching from "unipolar" to bipolar II. *Archives of General Psychiatry, 52,* 114–123.

Akiskal, H. S., Rosenthal, T. L., Haykal, R. F., Lemmi, H., Rosenthal, H. L., & Scott-Strauss, A. (1990) Characterological depression. *Archives of General Psychiatry, 37,* 777–786.

Boyce, P., Parker, J., Ravindran, A. V., Cooney, M., & Smith, F. (1991). Personality as a vulnerability factor to depression. *British Journal of Psychiatry, 159,* 100–114.

Davidson, J. R. T., France, R. D., Krishnan, R. R. K., & Pelton, S. (1985). Neurovegetative symptoms in chronic pain and depression. *Journal of Affective Disorders, 9,* 213–218.

Davidson, J. R. T., Giller, E. L., Zisook, S., & Overall, J. E. (1988a). An efficacy study of isocarboxazid and placebo in depression and its relationship to depressive nosology. *Archives of General Psychiatry, 45,* 120–128.

Davidson, J. R. T., Lipper, S., Pelton, S., Miller, R. D., Hammett, E., Mahorney, S. L., & Varia, I. (1988b). The response of depressed inpatients to isocarboxazid. *Journal of Clinical Psychopharmacology, 23,* 193–200.

Davidson, J. R. T., Miller, R. D., Turnbull, C. D., & Sullivan, J. L. (1982). Atypical depression. *Archives of General Psychiatry, 39,* 527–534.

Davidson, J. R. T., & Pelton, S. (1986). Forms of atypical depression and their response to antidepressants. *Psychiatry Research, 17,* 87–95.

Davidson, J. R. T., Pelton, S., Miller, R. D., & Lipper. S. (1986). Endogenous depression and the response to isocarboxazid. *Clinical Neuropharmacology, 9*(4), 563–565.

Davidson, J. R. T., Pelton, S., Woodbury, M., & Krishnan, R. R. K. (1988c). A study of depressive typology using Grade of Membership analysis. *Psychological Medicine, 18,* 179–189.

Davidson, J. R. T., & Raft, D. (1985). Monoamine oxidase inhibitors in patients with chronic pain. *Archives of General Psychiatry, 42,* 635–636.

Davidson, J. R. T., Raft, D., & Pelton, S. (1987). An outpatient evaluation of phenelzine and imipramine. *Journal of Clinical Psychiatry, 48,* 143–146.

Davidson, J. R. T., & Turnbull, C. D. (1984). The importance of dose in isocarboxazid therapy. *Journal of Clinical Psychiatry, 45*(7), 49–52.

Davidson, J. R. T., Zisook, S., Giller, E., & Helms, M. (1989a). Symptoms of interpersonal sensitivity in depression. *Comprehensive Psychiatry, 30,* 357–368.

Davidson, J. R. T., Zisook, S., Giller, E. L. Jr., & Helms, M. (1991). Predictors of response to monoamine oxidase inhibitors: Do they exist? *European Archives of Psychiatry and Clinical Neuroscience, 241,* 181–186.

Davidson, J. R. T., Zisook, S., Giller, E. L. Jr., & Woodbury, M. A. (1989b). Grade of membership analysis of depression: A confirmation study. *Psychological Medicine, 19,* 987–998.

Derogatis, L. R., Lipman, R. S., Rickels, K., & Covi, L. (1974). The Hopkins Symptom Checklist (HSCL): A self report inventory. *Behavioral Science, 19,* 1–15.

Hamilton, M. (1960). Rating scale for depression. *Journal of Neurology and Neurosurgical Psychiatry, 25,* 56–62.

Kiloh, L. G., Child, J. P., & Latner, G. (1959). A controlled trial of iproniazid in the treatment of endogenous depression. *Journal of Mental Science, 106,* 1139–1144.

Klein, D. F., Gittelman, R., Quitkin, F. M., & Rifkin, A. (1985). *Diagnosis and drug treatment of psychiatric disorders: Adults and children.* Baltimore: Williams & Wilkins.

Lascelles, R. G. (1965). Atypical facial pain and depression. *British Journal of Psychiatry, 112,* 651–659.

Liebowitz, M. R., Quitkin, F. M., Stewart, J. W., McGraber, P. J., Harrison, W., Rabkin, J., Tricamo, E., Markowitz, J. S., & Klein, D. F. (1984). Phenelzine vs imipramine in atypical depression. *Archives of General Psychiatry, 41,* 669–677.

Nierenberg, A. A., Pava, J. A., Clancy, K., Rosenbaum, J. F., & Fava, M. (1996). Are neurovegetative symptoms stable in relapsing or recurrent atypical depressive episodes? *Biological Psychiatry, 40,* 691–696.

McGrath, P. J., Stewart, J. W., Quitkin, F. M., Wager, S., Jenkins, S. W., Archibald, D. G., Stringfellow, J., & Robinson, D. S. (1994). Gepirone treatment of atypical depression: Preliminary evidence of serotonergic involvement. *Journal of Clinical Psychopharmacology, 14,* 347–352.

Nolen, W. A. (1986). Tranylcypromine in depression resistant to cyclic antidepressants. *Clinical Neuropharmacology, 9(4),* 569–571.

Pande, A. C., Birkett, M., Fechner-Bates, S., Haskett, R. F., & Greden, J. F. (1996). Fluoxetine versus phenelzine in atypical depression. *Biological Psychiatry, 40,* 1017–1020.

Paykel, E. S., Parker, R. R., Rowan, P. R., Rao, B. M., & Taylor, C. N. (1983). Nosology of atypical depression. *Psychological Medicine, 13,* 131–139.

Pollitt, J. (1965). Suggestions for a physiological classification of depression. *British Journal of Psychiatry, 111,* 489–495.

Raft, D., Davidson, J. R. T., Maltox, A., Mueller, R., & Wasik, J. (1979). A double-blind evaluation of phenelzine, amitriptyline and placebo in depression associated with pain. In T. Singer, R. Van Korff, & D. L. Murphy (Eds.), *Monoamine oxidase: Structure, function and altered functions* (pp. 507–516). New York: Academic Press.

Robinson, D. S., Kayser, A., Corcella, J., Larex, D., Yingling, K., & Howard, D. (1985). Panic attacks in outpatients with depression: Response to antidepressant treatment. *Psychopharmacology Bulletin, 21,* 562–567.

Sargant, W., & Dally, P. J. (1962). Treatment of anxiety states by antidepressant drugs. *British Medical Journal, 1,* 6–9.

Sargant, W., & Slater, E. (1972). *An introduction by physical methods of treatment in psychiatry.* New York: Science House.

West, E. D., & Dally, P. J. (1959). Effects of iproniazid in depressive syndromes. *British Medical Journal, 1,* 1491–1494.

CHAPTER 12

Chronic (and Hysteroid) Dysphorias

Jonathan W. Stewart
Donald F. Klein

This chapter documents pharmacological responsivity in chronic affective conditions variously referred to as hysteroid dysphoria, borderline personality, and chronic dysphoria.

Terminology and Conceptual Issues

Psychiatric nosology has labeled patients who chronically or intermittently experience dysphoric mood states as having depressive neurosis, depressive personality, or depressive character pathology. Such formulations accurately capture the long-standing, ingrained nature of the disorder but fail to emphasize that these disorders are treatable with antidepressant medication. Within this broad group of so-called characterologic depressions, Akiskal et al. (1980) identified a dysthymic subtype with sleep electroencephalographic characteristics of depressive disease. It was not until DSM-III (American Psychiatric Association, 1980) that the mood disorder of chronically depressed patients was made official by placing dysthymia among the mood disorders, a concept our group has attempted to underscore in the conceptualization of hysteroid dysphoria (Klein & Davis, 1969; Liebowitz & Klein, 1981), chronic dysphoria (Klein, 1974), and atypical depression (Liebowitz et al., 1984).

We present evidence that the chronic mood disorders rightly belong among the other affective disorders. This evidence comes mainly from our experience with psychopharmacological dissection studies but also from a family history study.

If a basic underlying mood disturbance is the foundation for the dysphoria of chronically depressed patients, standard antidepressant medications ought to be effective, and perhaps just as effective as for patients with more classical unipolar, episodic, or endogenomorphic depression. If character pathology or some mood-unrelated etiology accounts for chronic unhappiness, usual antidepressants should not be effective or should be substantially less effective for classical depressions.

Our hypothesis, then, is that antidepressant medications will be effective in the treatment of chronic depressions and that familial rates of depression will be as high in patients with chronic depression as in those with episodic depression. We present treatment studies of our own and a review of the literature.

Pharmacological Strategies

Study 1

In the first study (Liebowitz et al., 1988; Quitkin et al., 1988, 1989; Stewart et al., 1989), patients were 18–65 years of age, with a DSM-III diagnosis of either major depression or dysthymic disorder. None had melancholia. Prior to treatment, they reported whether they had been depressed all their life without significant well-being (chronic dysphoria), part of their life but at least half the time, or less than half the time. They were then randomly assigned after 1-week placebo washout to 6 weeks treatment with phenelzine, imipramine, or placebo. Phenelzine was pushed to 90 mg/day with mean final dose of 74 mg/day, imipramine was increased to 300 mg/day with mean dose of 254 mg/day, and maximum placebo was 6 pills/day. After 6 weeks of treatment, response was assessed by the treating psychiatrist's Clinical Global Impression Global Improvement rating of "much improved" or "very much improved." Patients who were "minimally improved," "unchanged," or "worse" were considered nonresponders. This is a conservative rating such that patients had to have improved at least 65% to be responders. Although other rating scale scores entirely corroborated the treating psychiatrist's judgment, only the percent response is shown.

Table 12.1 shows rate of response to each treatment according to baseline chronicity category. The perhaps unexpected outcome was that the high placebo response of the patients who were not chronically depressed resulted in failure to demonstrate efficacy of antidepressants in this population. More germane to our present topic, however, is that robust medication effects were seen both in patients with chronic dysphoria and

TABLE 12.1. Response by Illness Course

Illness course	Placebo	Imipramine	Phenelzine
Episodic	42% (9/21)	42% (5/12)	67 (8/12)
Other chronic depression	23% (15/64)	52% (38/73)	70% (57/82)
Chronic dysphoria	17% (9/52)	46% (22/48)	70% (37/53)

in other chronically depressed patients. Thus, even for patients who said they had been depressed their entire lives without significant periods of well-being, both imipramine and phenelzine were significantly more effective than was placebo. This clearly suggested that among chronically depressed outpatients, many can benefit dramatically from antidepressant medication.

Study 2

The second study (Stewart et al., 1996) investigated the efficacy of fluoxetine in depressed outpatients, again ages 18–65, who met DSM-III-R (American Psychiatric Association, 1987) criteria for major depression but without melancholia. Again, chronicity was rated at baseline as meeting criteria for chronic dysphoria, being chronic without chronic dysphoria, or being nonchronic. This was a 12-week open trial of fluoxetine 20 mg/day. After 12 weeks, those who were not rated as at least much improved had their dose raised to 40–80 mg/day by doctor's choice for an additional six weeks. Table 12.2 shows the results of this study. As with imipramine and phenelzine, the different categories of chronicity do not differ in rates of response to fluoxetine. If we include the patients who had their fluoxetine

TABLE 12.2. Response to Fluoxetine

Illness course	20 mg/day	> 20 mg/day	Total
Episodic	60% (29/48)	67% (10/15)	81% (39/48)
Other chronic depression	66% (25/38)	44% (4/9)	76% (29/38)
Chronic dysphoria	64% (63/948)	62% (18/29)	83% (81/98)

dose raised above 20 mg/day, the overall response rate to fluoxetine is 81%. Certainly, some of this improvement is nonspecific, as patients were continued on fluoxetine for 4½ months, but it is still impressive that more than 80% of a population of chronically depressed patients could so dramatically improve.

Literature Review

We wondered whether our experience on the efficacy of certain classes of antidepressants in chronic depression was unique or whether similar results had been reported in the literature. Table 12.3 summarizes the literature since 1980 on the pharmacological treatment of chronic depression. We found four studies in which patients were diagnosed as having neurotic depression, two of them placebo controlled (Banerji et al., 1989; Bohm et al., 1990; Taneri & Kohler, 1989; vander Velde, 1981). In all four studies, 60% or more of the patients improved with active medication, compared to less than one in five on placebo.

Six studies reported outcome for patients considered to have dysthymia but without major depression (Akiskal et al., 1980; Stewart et al., 1985; Stabl et al., 1989; Guelfi et al., 1989; Stewart et al., 1989; Kemali, 1989). Here, there was a 65% response to nontricyclics, almost half the patients responded to a tricyclic, and about one-quarter to placebo. Finally, in patients with major depression superimposed on dysthymia, so-called double depression (Keller & Shapiro, 1982), 80% responded to a nontricyclic, 60% to a tricyclic, and 19% to placebo (Harrison et al., 1986; Kocsis et al., 1988; Stewart et al., 1989). Clearly, by whatever definition of chronicity, and whether or not major depression is also present, chronically depressed patients improve with antidepressants.

TABLE 12.3. Literature Review of Pharmacological Treatment of Chronic Depression

	Non-TCA	TCA	Placebo
Neurotic depression (4 studies)	74% (81/110)	71% (54/75)	18% (6/33)
"Pure" dysthymia (6 studies)	65% (62/95)	48% (43/90)	25% (15/60)
Double depression (3 studies)	80% (16/20)	60% (25/42)	19% (8/43)

Note. TCA, tricyclic antidepressant.

Chronic Dysphorias and the Question of Borderline Personality

Parsons et al. (1989) reviewed the concept of borderline personality, concluding that it is a heterogeneous category. Patients with borderline personality have profound emotional instability, but there are definite differences between the schizotypal, those plagued by marked rejection sensitivity as in hysteroid dysphoria and those whose unstable, intense interpersonal relationships cause much volatile anger and aggressive behavior.

Parsons et al. (1989) reanalyzed data from the studies of Quitkin et al. (1988) comparing placebo, imipramine, and phenelzine in atypical depressives. They studied two consecutive groups of patients. In the first group of 171 patients, using the DSM-III borderline checklist, 23% had five or more symptoms and 33% had four or more. Using the five-feature criterion, 20% responded to placebo, 38% to imipramine, and 89% to phenelzine—a surprisingly positive phenelzine effect. If the definition is modified to include patients with four or more features, practically the same outcome proportions were found. A second set of 110 patients was rated by the Personality Assessment Form. A more stringent and a less stringent criterion were used with very little difference, the results being remarkably similar to the previous sample.

Amalgamating the entire sample and using the broader definitions, striking differences were found among treatment groups: 21% responded to placebo (8/38), 38% responded to imipramine (13/34), and 91% responded to phenelzine (20/22) ($\chi^2 = 28.3$, $p < .001$, $df = 2$). Imipramine was not significantly different from placebo, whereas phenelzine was much superior to both placebo and imipramine. In fact, comparing phenelzine with imipramine by borderline status indicated a negative effect of imipramine on borderline patients as compared to atypical depressives who did not have borderline features. This agrees with Klein's (1968) original report that imipramine produced anger in patients with emotionally unstable character disorder, and Soloff et al.'s (1986) report that amitriptyline caused increased hostility in a subset of patients with borderline personality disorder.

Borderline personality disorder and hysteroid dysphoria are overlapping but not identical concepts. Among atypical depressives, hysteroids were more than twice as likely to meet criteria for borderline personality as nonhysteroids. Of the atypical depressives, roughly 20% met criteria for hysteroid dysphoria and approximately 23% for borderline personality.

Despite the availability of research (Cowdry & Gardner, 1988) and clinical (Brinkley, 1993) reports on the utility of monoamine oxidase inhibitors (MAOIs) in borderline personality, there has been considerable reluctance to use these agents for such patients. We inform all our patients that a food-induced hypertensive crisis may result in a stroke or death and have been impressed that these patients take this warning quite seriously. Further, we now have the patients carry nifedipine with them to chew and swallow if they have a sudden throbbing occipital headache.

The recent development of reversible MAOIs, which do not cause hypersensitivity to tyramine, is extremely promising. It seems likely that this type of drug will be widely used for chronic atypical depression, hysteroid dysphoria, and borderline personality.

Discussion

These data begin to answer whether chronic depression belongs among the affective disorders. If it does, patients who report having been chronically depressed should respond in the same way to the standard pharmacological agents and should report the same familial rates of depression as do depressed patients who have been more episodically depressed. The pharmacological data presented suggest that the usual antidepressant medications are also effective for patients with chronic depression, and that they have relatively high rates of affective disorder in their families. This suggests that chronic depression rightly belongs among the affective disorders.

Such a conclusion is too glib and does not do the data proper justice, however. For example, tricyclic antidepressants are usually effective for at least 75% of patients with melancholia. Both our own work and the literature suggest that only 50–60% of nonmelancholic patients can be expected to improve with tricyclic antidepressants. Yet, these patients have a disorder highly responsive to somatic therapy, MAOIs and serotonin reuptake inhibitors being very effective. This different pattern of medication response—high tricyclic response in melancholics; more modest tricyclic response in chronic depressives coupled with high likelihood of response to other agents—suggests that patients with dysthymia might have a different disorder than do patients with melancholia. An unpublished family study from our group (Stewart, 1988) suggests that dysthymia and melancholia tend to breed true. If replicated, this would mean that some chronic depressive conditions and melancholia represent distinct disorders.

Conclusion

The data and the literature point toward chronic depression and melancholia as potentially separable disorders. Thus, chronic depression in general, and dysthymia in particular, might not be a subsyndromal variant of melancholia but rather a separate disorder in its own right. That the apparently more severe disorder responds better to imipramine than the lesser illness speaks for a qualitative distinction. Nevertheless, strategically, it seems best to maintain dysthymia and the other chronic depressive conditions within the rubric of the affective disorders because they are very treatable with standard antidepressant medications. This important treatment implication will be best highlighted by including categories for chronic depressive conditions among the affective disorders rather than with personality, character, or neurotic disorders.

Acknowledgment

This work was supported in part by U.S. Public Health Service Grants MH-30906 and MH-39143.

References

Akiskal, H. S., Rosenthal, T. L., Haykal, R. F., Lemmi, H., Rosenthal, R. H., & Scott-Strauss, A. (1980). Characterologic depressions: Clinical and sleep EEG findings separating "subaffective dysthymias" from "character-spectrum" disorders. *Archives of General Psychiatry, 37,* 777–783.

American Psychiatric Association. (1980). *Diagnostic and statistical manual of mental disorders* (3rd ed.). Washington, DC: Author.

American Psychiatric Association. (1987). *Diagnostic and statistical manual of mental disorders* (3rd ed., rev.). Washington, DC: Author.

Banerji, J. R., Brantingham, P., McEwan, G. D., Mason, J., Munt, D. F., Renton, R. L., Scott, A. P., Strakova, J. M., & Stevens, V. (1989). A comparison of alprazolam with amitriptyline in the treatment of patients with neurotic or reactive depression: A report of a randomized, double-blind study by a General Practitioner Working Party. *Irish Journal of Medical Science, 158,* 110–113.

Bohm, C., Robinson, D. S., & Gammans, R. E. (1990). Buspirone therapy in anxious elderly patients: A controlled clinical trial. *Journal of Clinical Psychopharmacology, 10,* 47S–51S.

Brinkley, J. R. (1993). Pharmacotherapy of borderline states. *Psychiatric Clinics of North America, 16,* 853–884.

Cowdry, R. W., & Gardner, D. L. (1988). Pharmacotherapy of borderline personality disorder. *Archives of General Psychiatry, 45,* 111–119.

Guelfi, J. D., Pichot, P., & Dreyfus, J. F. (1989). Efficacy of tianeptine in anxious-depressed patients: Results of a controlled multicenter trial versus amitriptyline. *Neuropsychobiology, 22,* 42–48.

Harrison, W., Rabkin, J., Stewart, J. W., McGrath, P. J., Tricamo, E., & Quitkin, F. (1986). Phenelzine for chronic depression: A study of continuation treatment. *Journal of Clinical Psychiatry, 47*, 346–349.

Keller, M. B., & Shapiro, R. W. (1982). "Double depression": Superimposition of acute depressive episodes on chronic depressive disorders. *American Journal of Psychiatry, 139*, 438–442.

Kemali, D. (1989). A multicenter Italian study of amineptine (survector 100). *Clinical Neuropharmacology, 12*(Suppl. 2), S41–S50.

Klein, D. F. (1968). Psychiatric diagnosis and a typology of clinical drug effects. *Psychopharmacologia, 13*, 359–386.

Klein, D. F. (1974). Endogenomorphic depression. *Archives of General Psychiatry, 31*, 447–454.

Klein, D. F., & Davis, J. (1969). *The diagnosis and drug treatment of psychiatric disorders.* Baltimore: Williams & Wilkins.

Kocsis, J. H., Frances, A. J., Voss, C., Mann, J. J., Mason, B. J., & Sweeney, J. (1988). Imipramine treatment for chronic depression. *Archives of General Psychiatry, 45*, 253–257.

Liebowitz, M. R., & Klein, D. F. (1981). Interrelationship of hysteroid dysphoria and borderline personality disorder. *Psychiatric Clinics of North America, 4*, 67–87.

Liebowitz, M. R., Quitkin, F. M., Stewart, J. W., McGrath, P. J., Harrison, W. M., Markowitz, J. S., Rabkin, J. G., Tricamo, E., Goetz, D. M., & Klein, D. F. (1988). Antidepressant specificity in atypical depression. *Archives of General Psychiatry, 45*, 129–137.

Liebowitz, M. R., Quitkin, F. M., Stewart, J. W., McGrath, P. J., Harrison, W., Rabkin, J., Tricamo, E., Markowitz, J. S., & Klein, D. F. (1984). Atypical depression. *Archives of General Psychiatry, 41*, 669–677.

Parsons, B., Quitkin, F. M., McGrath, P. J., Stewart, J. W., Tricamo, E., Ocepek-Welikson, K., Harrison, W., Rabkin, J. G., Wager, S. G., & Nunes, E. (1989). Phenelzine, imipramine and placebo in borderline patients meeting criteria for atypical depression. *Psychopharmacology Bulletin, 25*(4), 524–534.

Quitkin, F. M., McGrath, P. J., Stewart, J. W., Harrison, W., Wager, S. G., Nunes, E., Rabkin, R. G., Tricamo, E., Markowitz, J., & Klein, D. F. (1989). Phenelzine and imipramine in mood reactive depressives. *Archives of General Psychiatry, 46*, 787–793.

Quitkin, F. M., Stewart, J. W., McGrath, P. J., Liebowitz, M. R., Harrison, W. M., Tricamo, E., Klein, D. F., Rabkin, J. G., Markowitz, J. S., & Wager, S. G. (1988). Phenelzine versus imipramine in probable atypical depression: Defining syndrome boundaries of selective MAOI responders. *American Journal of Psychiatry, 145*, 306–312.

Soloff, P., George, A., Nathan, S., Schulz, P. M., Ulrich, R. F., & Perel, J. M. (1986). Progress in pharmacotherapy of borderline disorders. *Archives of General Psychiatry, 43*, 691–697.

Stabl, M., Biziére, K., Schmid-Burg, K. W., & Amrein, R. (1989). Review of comparative clinical trials: Moclobemide vs. tricyclic antidepressants and vs. placebo in depressive states. *Journal of Neural Transmission, 28*, 77–89.

Stewart, J. W. (1988). [A family history study of outpatient depression]. Unpublished manuscript, Columbia University, New York.

Stewart, J. W., McGrath, P. J., Liebowitz, M. R., Harrison, W., Quitkin, F., & Rabkin, J. G. (1985). Treatment outcome validation of DSM-III depressive subtypes: Clinical usefulness in outpatients with mild to moderate depression. *Archives of General Psychiatry, 42,* 1148–1153.

Stewart, J. W., McGrath, P. J., & Quitkin, F. M. (1996). [Fluoxetine response of depressed outpatients having varying degrees of chronicity]. Unpublished raw data.

Stewart, J. W., McGrath, P. J., Quitkin, F. M., Harrison, W., Markowitz, J., Wager, S., & Liebowitz, M. R. (1989). Relevance of DSM-III depression subtype and chronicity of antidepressant efficacy in atypical depression: Differential response to phenelzine, imipramine, and placebo. *Archives of General Psychiatry, 46,* 1080–1087.

Taneri, Z., & Kohler, R. (1989). Fluoxetine versus nomifensine in outpatients with neurotic or reactive depressive disorder. *International Clinical Psychopharmacology, 4*(Suppl. 1), 57–61.

vander Velde, C. (1981). Maprotiline versus imipramine and placebo in neurotic depression. *Journal of Clinical Psychiatry, 42,* 138–141.

CHAPTER 13

Minor and Recurrent Brief Depression

Jules Angst

This chapter describes forms of minor and intermittent depressive conditions that are not covered by classical conceptions of depression.

Criteria for Minor and Recurrent Brief Depression

The diagnostic concepts of minor depression and recurrent brief depression have been developed recently. As shown by reviews (Merikangas et al., 1996a, 1996b) for DSM-IV (American Psychiatric Association, 1994) there is a lack of data on these subtypes of depression. Minor depression was originally defined by Research Diagnostic Criteria (Spitzer et al., 1978) as an illness of at least 2 weeks' duration with sustained depressed mood. The RDC included both chronic and acute cases but excluded bereavement. The specific criteria required the presence of depressed mood and at least 2 of 16 symptoms, many of which comprise traits rather than episodic somatic symptoms. (An episode of 1 week is considered probable and 2 weeks' duration a definite minor depression.) In ICD-10, "mild depressive disorders" are equivalent to minor depression. Although the definition is given by the World Health Organization (1992), the term is not specifically included in ICD-10. Similarly, DSM-III (American Psychiatric Association, 1980) and DSM-III-R (American Psychiatric Association, 1987) do not include a formal definition of the concept of minor depression. Nevertheless, it would be logical to include a definition of minor depression as long as the term "major depression exists."

In an ongoing prospective epidemiological study of a cohort of the population from ages 20 to 30 in Zurich, Switzerland, two subtypes of affective disorders with no DSM-III-R or ICD-10 criteria provided substantial coverage of treated but undiagnosed cases of depression: minor depression and recurrent brief depression.

The DSM-III-R diagnostic criteria for major depression and the Zurich criteria for minor depression are given in Table 13.1. For a diagnosis of major depression, a minimal length of an episode of 2 weeks and the presence of at least five of nine criterial symptoms are required. Minor depression was defined in Zurich as a depressive episode of 2 weeks with only three or four of nine criterial symptoms. (Subjects with one or two of nine symptoms did not appear to be real cases in terms of the indicators of treatment and impairment.)

The third category, recurrent brief depression, requires the same number of depressive symptoms as major depression (four of eight of DSM-III or five of nine of DSM-III-R). In contrast to major depression, the episodes are brief (shorter than 14 days, usually 1 to 3 days) and must recur at least monthly over 1 year. In addition, subjective work impairment is required for case definition in epidemiological studies.

Design and Methods of the Zurich Study

The subjects for the study are those from the Zurich study, a longitudinal, epidemiological cohort study of young adults in Zurich, Switzerland (Angst et al., 1984). A cohort of 292 males and 299 females ages 19–20 years from the canton of Zurich was selected according to scores on the 90-item

TABLE 13.1. Diagnostic Criteria for Affective Subtypes

	Major depression (DSM-III-R)	Minor depression (Zurich)	Recurrent brief depression (Zurich)
Length of episode	Extended ≥ 2 weeks	Extended ≥ 2 weeks	Brief < 2 weeks
Frequency	nsp	nsp	At least monthly
Depressed mood	+	+	+
Number of criterial symptoms (DSM-III-R)	≥ 5/9	3 or 4/9	≥ 5/9
Subjective work impairment	nsp	nsp	Present

Note. nsp, not specified.

Hopkins Symptom Checklist (HSCL-90-R; Derogatis, 1977) in 1978. There were four waves of interviews over 10 years: 1979, 1981, 1986 and 1988. The interviews were carried out by well-trained clinical psychologists in the homes of the subjects and took about 3 hours each (Angst, 1995).

Prevalence Rates and Social Consequences

Application of the diagnostic criteria cited in Table 13.1 for minor depression in four interviews across 10 years yielded a weighted total lifetime prevalence rate (Table 13.2) at age 30 of minor depression of 11% (9.7% for males and 12.4% for females). These rates include cases of comorbidity.

This chapter focuses on the following mutually exclusive subgroups of depression: 37 "pure" cases of minor depression (i.e., those with no overlap with recurrent brief depression, major depression, or dysthymia) and 105 cases of recurrent brief depression. These two groups were compared to major depressive episodes and to controls ($n = 277$). Four cases with dysthymia alone and 28 cases that did not meet any of the criteria for depression yet had been treated were excluded from the analyses. Major depressive episodes took precedence over dysthymia; dysthymia took precedence over recurrent brief depression and the latter over minor depression.

The weighted lifetime prevalence rates at age 30 are (Table 13.3) pure minor depression, 7.8%; pure recurrent brief depression, 11.1%; pure major depression, 11.2%; and both major and recurrent brief depression, 4.9%.

TABLE 13.2. Sex-Specific Lifetime Rates for DSM-III-R Affective Subtypes (Not Mutually Exclusive)

	Males ($n = 292$)	Females ($n = 299$)	Males + females ($n = 591$)
Unweighted (%)			
Major depression	16.4	31.1	23.9
Recurrent brief depression	19.9	30.1	25.0
Dysthymia	4.8	3.7	4.2
Minor depression (all)	10.6	9.7	10.2
Weighted (%)			
Major depression	10.2	21.9	16.1
Recurrent brief depression	11.0	20.9	16.0
Dysthymia	1.9	2.4	2.2
Minor depression (all)	9.7	12.4	11.0

Note. Bipolars included.

TABLE 13.3. Prevalence and Sex Ratios of Depressive Subtypes (Mutually Exclusive Categories)

	Lifetime prevalence (%)	Female:male sex ratio
Minor depression	7.8	0.8
Recurrent brief depression	11.1	1.1
Major depression	11.2	1.5
Major + recurrent brief depression	4.9	3.5

The sex ratio is substantially different for minor depression than for major depression and recurrent brief depression. Whereas the sex ratio is almost equal for minor depression and recurrent brief depression, females exhibit significantly greater rates of major depression. Combined depression (i.e., major depression plus recurrent brief depression) is 3.5 times more frequent in females than in males.

A lifetime history of treatment of depression was present in 164 subjects. One-third to two-thirds of all subjects who met the criteria for one of the affective subtypes reported a history of treatment (Table 13.4): minor depression, 32%; recurrent brief depression, 50%; major depression, 41%; and major and recurrent brief depression, 71%.

Validity of the Diagnoses of Minor Depression and Recurrent Brief Depression

The validity of the affective subtypes of minor depression and recurrent brief depression was suggested by the high proportion of subjects with a history of treatment. In addition, the positive family history of depression

TABLE 13.4. Family History of Depression by Affective Subtypes

	Controls ($n = 277$)	MD ($n = 37$)	RBD ($n = 103$)	MDE ($n = 96$)	MDE + RBD ($n = 45$)	p
Lifetime history (%)						
Suicide attempts	2.5	2.7	13.6	15.6	33.3	.000
Treated depression	—	32.4	50.5	40.6	71.1	.000
Positive family history (%)						
Depression	33.7	54.6	63.2	56.6	71.4	.000
Treated depression	10.9	21.2	20.7	20.5	23.8	ns

Note. Bipolars included. MD, minor depression; RBD, recurrent brief depression; MDE, major depressive episode.

and treated depression was present twice as often among these depressive subgroups as among controls (Table 13.4).

Although the rate of suicide attempts over 10 years was low among minor depressives (2.7%), the rates of suicide attempts among recurrent brief depressives (13.6%) and major depressives (15.6%) were clearly elevated as compared to controls (2.5%) (Table 13.5). The highest rate of a history of suicide attempts was seen in the group suffering from both major depression and recurrent brief depression (33.3%).

Association with Other Psychiatric Syndromes

There was a high frequency of longitudinal overlap within the depressive subtypes (Angst & Hochstrasser, 1994). A history of minor depression was present in 10% of recurrent brief depressives, 8% of major depressives, and 7% of the combined group (Table 13.5). Over 10 years, dysthymia was diagnosed in 6% of minor depressives, 6% of recurrent brief depressives, 13% of major depressives, and 10% of the combined group.

A lifetime history of hypomania was found in equal proportions (i.e., 20%) of the minor depressives (odds ratio 3.7 [1.4–10.0]) and major depressives. However, no association was found between recurrent brief depression and hypomania (8.4%) compared to controls (6.8%). A lifetime history of social phobia was more frequently found among all groups of depressives. However, panic disorder was only associated with recurrent brief depression and major depression. Finally, the neurasthenic syndrome was three- to fourfold more frequent among recurrent brief and major depressives and twofold higher in minor depressives (odds ratio 2.4 [(1.0–5.5]) than in controls.

TABLE 13.5. Longitudinal Association of Affective Subtypes with Other Psychiatric Syndromes

	Controls (n = 277)	MD (n = 37)	RBD (n = 103)	MDE (n = 96)	MDE + RBD (n = 45)	p
Minor depression (%)	—	—	9.7	8.3	6.7	ns
Dysthymia (%)	—	6.1	5.6	13.1	9.5	.000
Hypomania (%)	6.8	20.0	8.4	17.2	26.7	.000
Social phobia (%)	2.5	8.1	14.6	13.5	13.3	.000
Agoraphobia (%)	4.0	5.4	7.8	13.5	13.3	.020
Panic disorder (%)	1.8	0.0	15.5	9.4	17.8	.000
Neurasthenia (%)	12.6	24.3	44.7	46.9	53.3	.000
Suicide attempts (%)	2.5	2.7	13.6	15.6	33.3	.000

Note. Bipolars included. MD, minor depression; RBD, recurrent brief depression; MDE, major depressive episode.

Course of Minor and Recurrent Brief Depression

The mean age of onset of depression was inversely related to the severity of the depressive subtype (minor depression, 17.6 ± 5.0 years; recurrent brief depression, 16.0 ± 4.75; major depression, 16.1 ± 4.98; recurrent brief depression + major depression, 15.0 ± 4.32).

The longitudinal course of minor depression was examined prospectively across the 10-year follow-up (1979-1988). Thirty-six of the 356 subjects who were interviewed at all four follow-ups met criteria for minor depression at age 20 or 22. (Figure 13.2). At follow-up in 1986 and 1988, the following findings emerged: 23 subjects (64%) did not suffer from a diagnosable depression; 13 (36%) once again received a diagnosis of depression, 4 of whom developed major depression; 7 had recurrent brief depression; and 2 had both subtypes. This suggests that minor depression is predictive of continued expression of depression in community subjects. However, most of the minor depressives developed more severe affective disorders over time.

The course of recurrent brief depression diagnosed at age 20 or 22 (1979, 1981) was also investigated (Figure 13.3). At follow-up in 1986 and 1988, 30 of the 56 cases (54%) did not suffer from a diagnosable depression; 16 cases (29%) received a diagnosis of recurrent brief depression again; and 13% developed into major depression and 4% into combined depression (major depression + recurrent brief depression).

The follow-up data of major depression (n = 52) in 1979 and 1981 (Figure 13.4) are also presented for comparative purposes: 46% did not receive a diagnosis during the follow-up period, 17% were diagnosed as pure major depression, and another 20% as major depression combined with other diagnoses. Therefore, 37% of major depressives received the same diagnosis again, and 15% developed into recurrent brief depression.

Conclusion

This chapter presents new operational definitions for both minor depression and recurrent brief depression using symptom criteria of DSM-III-R together with specific time criteria. A softer definition without duration criteria, as suggested by the work of Philipp et al. (1992) for patients from general practitioners, was not applied in our community sample in order to avoid too many false positives. We found a lifetime prevalence rate for minor depression at age 30 of 11%. This is compatible with the rate of 9.2% reported in another Swiss study carried out in Basle by Wacker et al. (1990), with 9.5% given by Maier et al. (1992) from Mainz, Germany, despite differences in the operational definitions across studies, and with 9.2% in the New Haven study of Weissman et al. (1978) applying RDC criteria.

The course of minor depression is distinct from recurrent brief depression in community samples: Whereas minor depression has a good prognosis in more than 60% of the cases, about 20% of the cases develop major depression and 20% recurrent brief depression.

In contrast, subjects with recurrent brief depression and major depression exhibit greater diagnostic stability over 6 to 8 years. Moreover, the longitudinal transition between these two subtypes is similar (i.e., 15–20%). In a comparison between the three affective subgroups, minor depression appears to fall between controls and recurrent brief depression in terms of severity, stability, sex ratio, and morbidity.

In summary, the use of the diagnostic category of minor depression helps to reduce the number of undiagnosed treated depressives. However, the remaining cases that meet diagnostic criteria for depression but do not receive treatment, and those that do receive treatment but do *not* meet criteria for a specific diagnostic subtype of depression (i.e., depression not otherwise specified) still need to be investigated.

Acknowledgments

This work was supported by Grant 3.873-0.88 from the Swiss National Science Foundation. I also thank Kathleen Ries Merikangas, PhD, Associate Professor of Psychiatry and Epidemiology, Director, Genetic Epidemiology Research Unit, Yale University, New Haven, Connecticut, for reviewing and advising the preparation of this chapter.

References

American Psychiatric Association. (1980). *Diagnostic and statistical manual of mental disorders* (3rd ed.). Washington, DC: Author.

American Psychiatric Association. (1987). *Diagnostic and statistical manual of mental disorders* (3rd ed., rev.). Washington, DC: Author.

American Psychiatric Association. (1994). *Diagnostic and statistical manual of mental disorders* (4th ed.). Washington, DC: Author.

Angst, J. (1995). Dépressions brèves récurrentes. In J. P. Olié, M. F. Poirier, H. Lôo (Eds.), *Les maladies dépressives* (pp. 223–233). Paris: Médecine Sciences Flammarion.

Angst, J., Dobler-Mikola, A., & Binder, J. (1984). The Zurich study. A prospective epidemiological study of depressive, neurotic and psychosomatic syndromes: I. Problem, methodology. *European Archives of Psychiatry and Neurological Sciences, 234,* 13–20.

Angst, J. & Hochstrasser, B. (1994). Recurrent brief depression: The Zurich Study. *Journal of Clinical Psychiatry, 55*(Suppl. 4), 3–9.

Derogatis, L. R. (1977). *Administration, scoring and procedures manual–II for the R (revised) version and other instruments of the Psychopathology Rating Scales Series.* Towson, MD: Leonard R. Derogatis.

Maier, W., Lichtermann, D., Oehrlein, A., & Fickinger, M. (1992). Depression in the community: A comparison of treated and non-treated cases in two non-referred samples. *Psychopharmacology, 106,* S79–81.

Merikangas, K. R., Ernst C., Maier, W., Hoyer, E. B. & Angst, J. (1996a) Minor depression. In T. A. Widiger, A. J. Frances, H. A. Pincus, R. Ross, M. B. First, & W. W. Davis (Eds.), *DSM-IV sourcebook* (Vol. 2, pp. 97–110). Washington, DC: American Psychiatric Association.

Merikangas, K. R., Hoyer, E. B., & Angst, J. (1996b). Recurrent brief depression. In T. A. Widiger, A. J. Frances, H. A. Pincus, R. Ross, M. B. First, & W. W. Davis (Eds.), *DSM-IV sourcebook* (Vol. 2, pp. 111–126). Washington, DC: American Psychiatric Association.

Philipp, M., Delmo, C. D., Buller, R., Schwarze, H., Winter, P., Maier, W., & Benkert, O. (1992). Differentiation between major and minor depression. *Psychopharmacology, 106,* S75–78.

Spitzer, R. L., Endicott, J., & Robins, E. (1978). Research diagnostic criteria: Rationale and reliability. *Archives of General Psychiatry, 35,* 773–782.

Wacker, H. R., Battegay, R., Mullejans, R., & Klein, K. H. (1990). *Prevalence of anxiety and mood disorders in a Swiss city.* Paper presented at CINP meeting, Kyoto, Japan.

Weissman, M. M., Myers, J. K., & Harding, P. S. (1978). Psychiatric disorder in a U.S. urban community 1975/76. *American Journal of Psychiatry, 135,* 459–462.

World Health Organization. (1992). *The ICD-10 classification of mental and behavioural disorders: Clinical descriptions and diagnostic guidelines.* Geneva: Author.

CHAPTER 14

Suicide in Chronic and Recurrent Depressions
Stuart A. Montgomery

Suicide is a relatively rare event occurring in the United Kingdom, for example, at the rate of 9 per 100,000 population annually. However, the risk of death from suicide is substantially raised in depressive illness. The rate of suicide or accidental death (some of which may have been suicide) in a depressed group was reported to be more than 4 times that of a control group of surgical patients (Tsuang et al., 1980); in another study it was reported to be raised by as much as 13 times compared with the general population (Hagnell et al., 1982). Estimates of approximately 15% of depressives who eventually kill themselves have been consistently reported (Guze & Robins, 1970). Based on such studies, it is further estimated that 1% of depressives die annually from suicide.

Large patient samples are needed to obtain valid estimates of events that occur at this frequency, and in small studies varying rates may by chance be observed. However, in some small studies even though no deaths were recorded, the rate of suicide attempts was clearly elevated. For example, Shapiro and Keller (1981) reported that 10% of their sample of 100 depressed patients had made a suicide attempt within the year of follow-up.

Chronicity and Suicide

Despite decades of research we lack reliable and specific predictors of suicide. Certain common features have been identified in groups of suicide attempters; for example, older, socially isolated males are more likely to make a suicide attempt. However, predictor scales developed from this type of observation can only give an estimate of increased risk; they are too imprecise to be able to identify the individual depressed patient who is likely to commit suicide.

The effect of the introduction of antidepressants on the suicide rate in depressed patients is difficult to assess without long-term studies that control for differences in patient history and treatment. For example, Avery and Winokur (1976), comparing the outcome of different management in depressed patients, found fewer suicides at follow-up associated with electroconvulsive therapy (ECT) than in patients who received inadequate or no treatment, though a higher rate was seen in patients who received antidepressants plus ECT. However, the selection bias inherent in the study, with more severe patients being allocated to the combined treatment, makes interpretation of the results difficult.

It is apparent that the risk of suicide increases in inadequately treated patients, and this suggestion is supported by the reports that only a minority of depressed patients who kill themselves are found to have received adequate antidepressant treatment (Modestin, 1985; Roy, 1982). Similar proportions are reported in those who make an unsuccessful suicide attempt (Prescott & Highley, 1985).

This lack of adequate treatment, worrisome in itself, reflects only one aspect of the undertreatment of depression. The epidemiological studies in both the United States and Europe have found that the majority of individuals who suffer from major depression do not seek treatment (Robins & Regier, 1990; Hurry et al., 1987). It is also unfortunate that depression is recognized in only half of those who do consult their primary care physician (Freeling et al., 1985). Because depression is associated with an increased suicide risk, failure to treat is likely to lead to the depressed individual spending longer periods at risk.

The length of time that those who suffer from major depression spend during episodes is in any case substantial. Depression is a long-term illness that is recurrent in the majority of cases. Early estimates of the percentage that are recurrent have had to be revised upwards, as studies with longer follow-up periods have shown recurrence rates of at least 70% (Angst, 1992b). A considerable amount of time, estimated at 20%, is spent in depressive episodes during a sufferer's lifetime, and the exposure to risk of suicide is therefore also high.

Repeat Suicidal Behavior and Recurrent Brief Depression

A link between depressive episodes and suicide attempts, identified in patients suffering from brief episodes of depression, has made an important contribution to our understanding of the phenomenon. The studies in which this link is detected were prospective investigations of the prophylactic efficacy of pharmacological treatment in reducing suicide attempts in patients with a history of repeated suicidal behavior. Major depression was an exclusion criterion in these studies that compared the prophylactic efficacy of both a low-dose neuroleptic (flupenthixol) and an antidepressant (mianserin) with placebo (Montgomery et al., 1979, 1983).

In spite of the exclusion of patients with major depression, it was found that during the 6-month study patients suffered brief episodes of depression that fulfilled the symptomatic criteria for major depression but lasted less than 2 weeks. Suicidal behavior appeared to be related to these episodes and at 4 weeks the depression score, rated on the Montgomery–Asberg Depression Rating Scale (MADRS; Montgomery & Asberg, 1979), was a significant predictor of subsequent suicide attempts. In addition to the total MADRS score, six of the individual items were also significant predictors of subsequent suicide attempts (Montgomery et al., 1983).

In subsequent studies following up a similar group of patients, the nature of these brief depressive episodes was investigated. The episodes appeared the same as major depression in symptoms and severity; they fulfilled DSM-III-R (American Psychiatric Association, 1987) criteria for major depression except that they did not last long enough to meet the 2-week minimum duration criterion. Two-thirds of the episodes lasted between 2 and 4 days, with a median of 3 days (Montgomery et al., 1989, 1990). Approximately 80% of the episodes lasted less than 5 days and 97% less than 1 week.

The brief episodes recurred with a median interval of 18 days from the start of one to the start of the next episode. They did not, however, recur at regular intervals, and the recurrence is best described as irregularly regular. Roughly equal numbers of intervals were recorded between 1 and 5 weeks and a median number of 20 episodes per year would be expected.

Severity of Recurrent Brief Depression

In spite of the brevity of the episodes, this is not a mild phenomenon. The mean severity of the episodes was 30 measured on the MADRS and two-thirds reached a score of 24 or more. This score is sometimes used to identify those who suffer moderate or severe depression for inclusion in efficacy studies of major depression. Twenty-five percent of the episodes had a score greater than 35 which is used to define severe depression.

The epidemiological studies of recurrent brief depression carried out by Angst and Dobler-Mikola (1985) in a normal population cohort study in Zurich reported that recurrent brief depression was common with an incidence at least as high as major depression. These studies did not have a clinical rating of severity of the episodes, but the criterion for an episode was social or occupational impairment.

Dysthymia and Recurrent Brief Depression

Some patients who suffer from recurrent brief depression may be mistakenly diagnosed as dysthymic, despite dysthymia's classification as a minor or mild condition. To fulfill the DSM-III-R or DSM-IV (American Psychiatric Association, 1994) diagnostic criteria for dysthymia, depression has to have been present for 2 years for most of the time. The reliability of memory over such a lengthy period is doubtful, and there is a tendency for those with recurrent episodes of depression that occur frequently but are of short duration to coalesce episodes in retrospect. The result is that what were discrete episodes appear in retrospect to be more chronic and to have lasted longer than was the case.

This type of factor may explain in part the high prevalence of pure dysthymia (1.7%) reported in the Epidemiologic Catchment Area study carried out in the United States which used retrospective reporting (Burke et al., 1988). Considerably lower rates are reported in prospectively gathered data. For example, in the Zurich study the lifetime prevalence of dysthymia was reported as 0.9% (Angst, 1992b).

Pure dysthymia (i.e., without comorbid major depression) is relatively uncommon compared with major depression or recurrent brief depression, but there is a group in which the conditions overlap. Most studies of the effectiveness of treatment in dysthymia have been conducted in patients who suffered from dysthymia and major depression or double depression. There is some overlap between dysthymia and recurrent brief depression, but this is more modest than the association with major depression. For instance, the odds ratio of an association between recurrent brief depression and dysthymia is reported as 2.6 by Angst (1990), compared to the odds ratio for major depression and dysthymia of 8.1. A study conducted in primary care which found an overlap with dysthymia in only 14 of 73 patients supports the view that recurrent brief depression is a separate disorder (Weiller et al., 1994).

Suicide and Recurrent Brief Depression

The link between suicide attempts and brief depressive episodes is important. In the clinical follow-up studies, attempts occurred only during episodes and not during the intervals between (Montgomery et al., 1989).

One explanation of the relationship between recurrent brief depression and suicide attempts could be that it is an artifact of patient selection in the clinical studies. However, the same link is also seen in the epidemiological studies of Angst (1990). A raised level of suicide attempts in the major depression group compared with the normal population was reported, as would be expected, and there was also a raised level in the recurrent brief depression group. There were more suicide attempts in the recurrent brief depression group than in major depression, although the numbers were too small for valid comparison.

A raised suicide attempt rate is perhaps not surprising in recurrent brief depression with its rapid onset and rapid resolution of episodes. The unpredictability of the episodes with rapid shifts from normal mood to deep depression are reported by sufferers to be very difficult to tolerate. Recurrent brief depression appears to be a stable illness persisting over many years, and the amount of time that those with recurrent brief depression may spend in depressive episodes may contribute to the increased risk of suicide attempts. In the clinical sample reported by Montgomery et al. (1989), a mean of 20% of the time is spent in episodes, which is very similar to the report of 20% of the time spent in episodes of major depression (Angst, 1992b).

Combined Conditions

An important extra factor contributing to an increase in the suicide attempt rate appears to be the comorbidity of recurrent brief depression with major depression. In both the epidemiological and the clinical studies there is a group of patients who suffer from both recurrent brief depression and major depression, termed "combined depression." In the clinical sample it has been observed that a patient who suffers from recurrent brief depression in whom a major depressive episode occurs, reverts on resolution of the major depression to the original pattern of brief episodes.

This group appears to be particularly at risk for suicide attempts compared with those with either condition alone. The epidemiological studies have found that although the suicide attempt rate is elevated in both recurrent brief depression and major depression in those who have the combined condition, the risk is increased threefold over either condition alone. In the 10-year community follow-up, one-third of the combined depression group reported a suicide attempt by the age of 30. The epidemiological studies in Zurich have also reported that there is a higher incidence of suicide attempts in the patients who suffer from dysthymia and major depression (Angst, 1992b).

Conclusion

Suicide and suicide attempts are regarded as the most serious and unfortunate consequences of depression, and it is important for clinicians to take into account the clinical and epidemiological data when assessing the risks for the individual. It is clear from this review that identifying sufferers from recurrent brief depression would improve our ability to spot those at a higher than normal risk of suicide or suicide attempts. Unfortunately, many patients with recurrent brief attacks of depression are often given the controversial label "borderline personality disorder," obscuring the link of these brief attacks to major affective episodes.

It is apparent that individuals who suffer from comorbid depressive states are at a substantially raised risk over those with simple major or recurrent brief depression alone. Those with combined depression (comorbid major and recurrent brief depression) and double depression (comorbid major depression and dysthymia) form a group with a very high risk of suicide attempts, and the clinician should take the greatest possible care in the management of these two groups. Suicide prevention efforts in chronic depressive disorders should be geared to the brief recurrent depressions interspersed between major depressive episodes.

References

Angst, A. (1990). Recurrent brief depression: A new concept of depression. *Pharmacopsychiatry, 23,* 63–66.

Angst, A. (1992a). Comorbidity of recurrent brief depression. *Clinical Neuropharmacology, 15*(Suppl. 1), 9–10.

Angst, A. (1992b). How recurrent and predictable is depressive illness? In S. A. Montgomery & F. Rouillon (Eds.), *Long-term treatment of depression* (pp. 1–14). Chichester: Wiley.

Angst, A., & Dober-Mikola, A. (1985). The Zurich Study IV. Recurrent and nonrecurrent brief depression. *European Archives of Psychiatry and Neurological Science, 234,* 30–37.

Avery, D., & Winokur, G. (1976). Mortality in depressed patients treated with electroconvulsive therapy and antidepressants. *Archives of General Psychiatry, 33,* 1029–1037.

Burke, J. D., Regier, D. A., & Christie, K. A. (1988). Epidemiology of depression: Recent findings from the NIMH epidemiologic catchment area program. In J. A. Swinkeels & W. Blijleven (Eds.), *Depression, anxiety and aggression* (pp. 23–28). Houten: Medidact.

Freeling, P., Rao, B. M., Paykel, E. S., Sireling, L. I., & Burton, R. H. (1985). Unrecognized depression in general practice. *British Medical Journal, 290,* 1880–1883.

Guze, S. B., & Robins, E. (1970). Suicide among primary affective disorders. *British Journal of Psychiatry, 117,* 437–438.

Hagnell, O., Lanke, J., Rorsman, B., & Ojesjo, L. (1982). Are we entering an age of melancholy? Depressive illness in a prospective epidemiological study over 25 years. The Lundby Study, Sweden. *Psychological Medicine, 12,* 279–289.

Hurry, J., Bebbington, P. E., & Tennant, C. (1987). Psychiatric symptoms and social disablement as determinants of illness behaviour. *Australian and New Zealand Journal of Psychiatry, 21,* 68–74.

Modestin, J. (1985). Antidepressant therapy in depressed clinical suicides. *Acta Psychiatria Scandinavica, 71,* 11–116.

Montgomery, S. A., & Asberg, D. (1979). A new depression scale designed to be more sensitive to change. *British Journal of Psychiatry, 134,* 382–389.

Montgomery, S. A., Montgomery, D., Baldwin, D., & Green, M. (1989). Intermittent 3-day depressions and suicidal behaviour. *Neuropsychobiology, 22,* 128–134.

Montgomery, S. A., Montgomery, D., Baldwin, D., & Green, M. (1990). The duration, nature and recurrence rate of brief depression. *Neuropsychopharmacology and Biological Psychiatry, 14,* 729–735.

Montgomery, S. A., Montgomery, D., Rani, J., Roy, D., Shaw, P. & McAuley, R. (1979). Maintenance therapy in repeat suicidal behaviour: A placebo controlled trial. *Proceedings of 10th International Congress for Suicide Prevention and Crisis Intervention,* pp. 227–229.

Montgomery, S. A., Roy, D., & Montgomery, D. (1983). The prevention of recurrent suicidal acts. *British Journal of Pharmacology, 15,* 183S–188S.

Prescott, L. F., & Highley, M. S. (1985). Drugs prescribed for self poisoners. *British Medical Journal, 290,* 1633–1636.

Robins, L. N., & Regier, D. A. (1990). *Psychiatric disorders in America: The epidemiologic catchment area study.* New York: Free Press.

Roy, A. (1982). Risk factors for suicide in psychiatric patients. *Archives of General Psychiatry, 39,* 1089–1095.

Shapiro, R. W., & Keller, M. B. (1981). Initial 6-month follow-up of patients with major depressive disorder. *Journal of Affective Disorders, 3,* 205–220.

Tsuang, M. T., Woolson, J. R. F., & Fleming, J. A. (1980). Premature deaths in schizophrenia and affective disorders. *Archives of General Psychiatry, 37,* 979–983.

Weiller, E., Boyer, P. Lépine, J.-P., & Lecoubier, Y. (1994). Prevalence of recurrent brief depression in primary care. *European Archives of Psychiatry and Clinical Neuroscience, 244,* 174–181.

CHAPTER 15

Depression and Attention-Deficit/ Hyperactivity Disorder

Rachel G. Klein

Because attention-deficit/hyperactivity disorder (ADHD) is believed to be related to depressive disorders, this chapter examines the familial and longitudinal course of ADHD, with specific focus on depression. ADHD is the most common childhood psychiatric disorder among clinical referrals in the United States. In spite of the fact that the diagnosis is not recognized in Europe, a high frequency of the disorder is most likely there as well. Although children with the disorder display excessive motor activity, the symptoms that bring them to professional attention are typically those associated with poor impulse control (disruptive, intrusive, attention-seeking behaviors) and impaired attention (failure to follow through on instructions and initiated tasks). Attention is a complex human function, with multiple components, each probably with its own regulatory processes that can become dysregulated. In children with ADHD, it is not the orienting aspect of attention that is dysfunctional but the maintenance of attention once it is engaged. ADHD children's attention can be readily; however, there is a low threshold for interference with sustained attentional effort, so that failure to complete initiated activities is typical. Usually, the child starts many tasks, turns from one to the other, and finishes none.

Although poor concentration is not an essential diagnostic feature of major depression, it is a very common feature of the disorder. However, the clinical nature of the attentional defect seems to differ between major depressive disorder and ADHD. In major depressive disorder, there seems to be impairment of orienting attention possibly due to loss of interest. In addition, there often is impairment of sustained attention, but individuals with major depression typically do not shift from one activity to another. If anything, the rough descriptive picture of inattention in ADHD resembles that found in mania rather than in major depression.

There are other important clinical differences between ADHD and major depression. The age of onset of ADHD is always in early childhood, typically toddlerhood. It is a chronic condition through childhood and early adolescence, and often remits during mid to late adolescence. There is a great preponderance of males among children with ADHD, with a male to female ratio of about 10 to 1 in clinical populations. In contrast, major depression is relatively rare in early childhood but soars in adolescence—a pattern of incidence that bears no resemblance to ADHD. The gender ratio for major depression seems to be even in childhood but shifts in adolescence with a disproportionate frequency of females. These clinical observations do not suggest a relationship between childhood ADHD and major depressive disorder. However, epidemiological, clinical, and familial studies of psychiatric disorders have linked the two conditions (Biederman et al., 1991, 1995; Cohen et al., 1993).

Clinical Studies of ADHD and Major Depressive Disorder in Children

Carlson and Cantwell (1980) reported that symptoms of depression were very common among children referred for behavioral problems. These are illustrated in Table 15.1. The authors note that depressive symptomatology is unsuspected in these children because of failure to conduct systematic inquiry concerning their presence (Carlson & Cantwell, 1980). The report indicates symptom frequency but not the rate of major depression in the behavior-disordered children whose diagnosis is unspecified. Therefore,

TABLE 15.1. Rates of Depressive Symptoms in 7- to 17-Year-Olds with Behavior Disorders (n = 27)

Symptom	Rate
Dysphoric mood	37%
Low self-esteem	44%
Anhedonia	37%
Fatigue	19%
Somatic complaints	30%
Suicidal ideation	37%
Hopelessness	37%

Note. Data are from Carlson and Cantwell (1980).

the degree of comorbidity between ADHD and major depression is unclear.

A relationship between depression and behavioral disorders was also noted by Puig-Antich (1982), who reported a high rate of major depression in children with conduct disorders. Because ADHD almost always accompanies conduct disorders in preadolescence, it is likely that the cases in the Puig-Antich study also had ADHD. Puig-Antich posited a specific causal relationship between major depressive disorder and conduct disorder. He argued that conduct disorders were secondary complications of the depressive disorders because treatment of the latter with tricyclic antidepressants ameliorated both sets of symptoms. However, tricyclics may be effective in children with behavioral disorders who are free of depression; therefore, a straightforward interpretation of treatment outcome is not evident (Puig-Antich & Gittelman, 1982). The lack of a control treatment condition further limits drawing inferences bearing on the relationship between the coexisting disorders.

Others have reported that at least a quarter of children with ADHD or hyperactivity in clinical settings meet criteria for major depression (Alessi & Magen, 1988; Biederman et al., 1987; Staton & Brumback, 1981). High comorbidity between major depression and ADHD has also been found in epidemiological studies (Anderson et al., 1987; Bird et al., 1988). In fact, in a large population study of 9-year-olds in New Zealand, major depression almost never occurred without another diagnosis, and 57% of those with major depressive disorder were diagnosed as having ADHD as well.

The clinical and epidemiological reports document a significant overlap between major depressive disorder and ADHD in young age.

Familial Association between ADHD and Major Depressive Disorder

Two investigative strategies have studied the association between ADHD and major depressive disorder in related individuals. One reports the psychiatric disorders in first-degree relatives of children with ADHD; the other reports on the status of children of adults with major depressive disorder.

In an attempt to elucidate whether ADHD represents a childhood variant of adult bipolar disease, Stewart and Morrison (1973) investigated the presence of affective disorders in the families of hyperactive (ADHD) children and medical controls. In addition, a sample of adopted hyperactive children was included. Not only was there no difference across the three groups in lifetime prevalence of affective disorder (unipolar and bipolar) in relatives, but absolute rates were low (6% to 10% for unipolar depression). This early report was influential, and for the ensuing decade it was assumed that there was no relationship between depression and hyperactivity.

Findings obtained by Lahey et al. (1988) are consistent with the above report. In a study of outpatients, the rate of major depression did not differ between parents of children with ADHD and parents of psychiatric controls. In contrast, mothers, but not fathers, of children with conduct disorders had significantly higher rates of major depression than did mothers of children with ADHD and mothers of controls. Therefore, it was the presence of antisocial disorders in the child, rather than the ADHD, that was correlated with an increase in major depression in mothers. However, this specific diagnostic relationship was not corroborated in another small outpatient study (Schachar & Wachsmuth, 1990).

Unlike the above investigators, Biederman et al. (1986, 1987) found an excess of major depression in first-degree relatives of a small group of children with ADD (many with ADHD) compared to relatives of pediatric controls. Rates for specific groups of relatives (e.g., mother, father, and sibling) are not specified in this study. The association between childhood ADD and familial major depressive disorder was unaffected by the presence of major depression in the children. In other words, the increase of major depressive disorder in relatives of ADD children was not due to the coexistence of an affective disorder in the index ADD children. In a subsequent large study, Biederman et al. (1990) replicated their earlier findings of a familial link between childhood ADD and major depressive disorder in first-degree relatives.

We have completed two large family studies of lifetime psychiatric history in parents of children with ADHD compared to parents of normal controls (Klein & Mannuzza, 1990). Because only a third of fathers were interviewed directly, the discussion is restricted to data on mothers. No excess of major depression was found in either study in mothers of children with ADHD and mothers of matched controls (see Table 15.2 for a summary of findings). The studies differ methodologically from others in that parents were interviewed at a time when their child was followed up in late adolescence/early adulthood (range = 16–23 years, mean = 18 years). In our investigations, children were diagnosed at mean age 9 (range = 6–13 years) and parents were interviewed about themselves about 10 years later. In other studies, parents were interviewed at the time the child was an identified patient. It is conceivable that parent self-reports are affected by the current clinical status of their child. That such may be the case is suggested by our findings that at the time we diagnosed the children, about 40% of parents retrospectively reported having had ADHD in childhood. However, the self-reported rate dropped dramatically to 5% when the

TABLE 15.2. Rates of Major Depression in Relatives of Children with ADHD

| | | Child diagnostic group | | | |
| | | 1 | 2 | 3 | |
Author	Relative[a]	ADHD (n)	Normal controls (n)	Patient controls (n)	p
Stewart &	M	3.4% (59)	4.9% (41)	— —	ns
Morrison (1973)	F	0% (59)	0% (41)	— —	ns
Biederman et al. (1987)	1st°	27% (20)	6% (15)	— —	.05
Lahey et al. (1988)	M	22% (18)	17% (30)	50% (14[b])	1 vs. 2, ns
	F	11%	17%		1 vs. 3 = .05
Biederman et al. (1990)	1st°	25% (73)	13.6% (26)	3.6% (26)	1 vs. 2, ns
					1 vs. 3 = .01
Klein & Mannuzza (1990)	M	16% (95)	19% (100)	— —	ns
Klein & Mannuzza (1990)	M	26% (73)	22% (64)	— —	ns

[a]M, mothers; F, fathers; 1st°, first-degree relatives.
[b]Conduct disorders.

parents were interviewed 10 years later, when their child was no longer in treatment. This methodological issue greatly complicates a clear understanding of results from studies of familial aggregation in affected children.

Because family studies are inconsistent in documenting an association between ADHD and major depression, it would be instructive to examine offspring of adults with major depression for any evidence of ADHD.

Such studies tend to focus on children's major depressive disorder and anxiety disorders; few indicate the prevalence of ADHD (see Table 15.3). In a careful study, Orvaschel et al. (1988) found a higher prevalence of

TABLE 15.3. Rates of ADHD in Offspring of Parents with Major Depression

| | Parent group | | | | |
Author	Major depression	(n)	Controls	(n)	p
Orvaschel et al. (1988)	19.7%	(61)	6.5%	(45)	.05
McClellan et al. (1990)	29%	(56)	6%	(47)	.001
Hammen (1991)	9%	(22)	8%	(38)	ns

Note. (n), number of children.

ADHD in the children of adults with depression than in those of normals. Similar results have been noted by Keller et al. (1988) and McClellan et al. (1990). In contrast, a low frequency of ADHD was found by Hammen (1991). The initial cross-sectional findings were confirmed in yearly reassessments over a 3-year period.

Problematically depressed mothers have reported more behavioral problems in their children than have nondepressed mothers (Breslau et al., 1988). It is difficult to assess to what extent the mothers' psychiatric history may have influenced their report of the child's functioning. In the absence of teacher reports, the diagnosis of ADHD based solely on parental reports is questionable. The study by Orvaschel et al. (1988) is the only one that reports findings on teacher ratings of classroom behavior. Children who were diagnosed as ADD were rated significantly more active and inattentive than were controls. Unfortunately, the report does not indicate whether teacher ratings of ADD children reached threshold for confirmation of the diagnosis. In Hammen's (1991) study, the school behavior ratings of children of depressed women were worse than those of controls, but the specific behavioral content is not reported. Problematically, ADD in these studies is as frequent in girls as it is in boys. This gender distribution is strikingly at variance with established findings for the disorder.

Longitudinal Studies of Children with ADHD

If, indeed, there is true comorbidity between major depression and ADHD, compared to non-ADHD children, children with ADHD should be at significantly higher risk for major depressive disorder as time progresses. Longitudinal studies are especially appropriate to address such questions because they are uniquely suited to the detection of new disorders. Several cohorts of children with ADHD have been followed into adolescence, and a couple into adulthood (Klein & Mannuzza, 1991; Mannuzza et al., 1993). None has found a higher rate of major depression in former hyperactive children either in adolescence or in adulthood, compared to controls. These results are extremely consistent. Findings from our own studies are presented in Tables 15.4 and 15.5.

Prospective follow-up studies have generated remarkably consistent findings that fail to support a link between ADHD and major depressive disorder. Because ADHD is much more common in boys than in girls, studies have been restricted to boys. The picture for girls might differ. We followed up the only cohort of girls with ADHD. It is small, totaling only 17 cases (vs. 200 boys), because of the rarity of the disorder in girls. In late adolescence (mean age 18), the rate of major depression in the girls was 12%, no different from 8% in a matched group of boys with ADHD. The

TABLE 15.4. Lifetime Rate of Major Depression in 16- to 23-Year-Old Adolescents Who Had ADHD as Children

	Child group				
Author	ADHD	(*n*)	Controls	(*n*)	*p*
Gittelman et al. (1985)	3%	(101)	10%	(100)	ns
Mannuzza et al. (1991)	7%	(94)	13%	(78)	ns

12% rate is not greater than what has been reported in population studies of female adolescents (Lewinsohn et al., 1993) and does not appear to indicate a specific vulnerability to major depression in women with an early history of ADHD.

The long-term follow-up studies provide a consistently negative body of data concerning to the relationship between ADHD and major depression.

Conclusion

The clinical studies suggest that a relatively large number of children with major depressive disorder also have ADHD. Comorbidity between the two conditions is less marked if one selects for ADHD, but it still is maintained. Family studies of relatives of children with ADHD have yielded conflicting results. It is possible that parents' reports of their own psychiatric history are affected by their coinciding with treatment of their child, because two large studies, conducted years after the children were diagnosed, and after the condition had remitted in the majority, obtained negative results. However, discrepant findings at the two points in time do not indicate which report is accurate. The fact that longitudinal studies of children with ADHD all fail to find an elevated risk for major depression in the children is a major problem for establishing the principle that ADHD and major depressive disorder are linked disorders, a theory that has implications for

TABLE 15.5. Rates of Major Depression in 23- to 30-Year-Old Adults Who Had ADHD as Children

Major depression	ADHD (*n* = 91)	Controls (*n* = 95)	*p*
Current	2%	0%	ns
Lifetime	23%	25%	ns

Note. Data are from Mannuzza et al. (1993).

diagnosis, treatment, and genetic studies of ADHD. Moreover, the fact that girls and boys are equally frequent among offspring of parents with depression raises questions concerning the equivalence of the ADHD syndrome between these cases and clinical referrals for ADHD.

Nevertheless, the positive relationship between affective and attention-deficit disorders observed in several sets of studies cannot be dismissed. One possibility is that children of adults with major depressive disorders have behavioral syndromes that represent a phenocopy of ADHD. To evaluate this hypothesis further, one would need to know ages of onset and course of offspring identified as ADHD to examine whether they follow patterns found in clinical cases of ADHD. If so, the challenge would remain concerning the lack of major depressive disorder in long-term outcome of hyperactive children. If not, the likelihood of phenocopies of ADHD in families of depressed adults should be considered.

Editors' note: It would be useful to study the relationship between ADHD and childhood onset bipolarity (Biederman et al., 1996).

References

Alessi, N. E., & Magen, J. (1988). Comorbidity of other psychiatric disturbances in depressed, psychiatrically hospitalized children. *American Journal of Psychiatry, 145,* 1582–1584.

Anderson, J. C., Williams, S., McGee, R., & Silva, P. A. (1987). DSM-III disorders in preadolescent children: Prevalence in a large sample from the general population. *Archives of General Psychiatry, 44,* 69–76.

Biederman, J., Faraone, S. V., Deenan, K., Knee, D., & Tsuang, M. T. (1990). Family-genetic and psychosocial risk factors in DSM-III attention deficit disorder. *Journal of the American Academy of Child and Adolescent Psychiatry, 29,* 526–533.

Biederman, J., Faraone, S., Mick, E., & Lelon, E. (1995). Psychiatric comorbidity among referred juveniles with major depression: Fact of artifact? *Journal of the American Academy of Child and Adolescent Psychiatry, 34,* 579–590.

Biederman, J., Faraone, S., Mick, E., Wozniak, J., Chen, L., Ouellette, C., Maris, A., Moore, P., Garcia, J., Mennin, D., & Lelon, E. (1996). Attention deficit hyperactivity disorder and juvenile mania: An overlooked comorbidity? *Journal of the American Academy of Child and Adolescent Psychiatry, 35,* 997–1008.

Biederman, J., Munir, K., Knee, D., Armentano, M., Autor, S., Hoge, S. K., Waternaux, C., & Tsuang, M. (1987). High rate of affective disorders in probands with attention deficit disorder and in their relatives: A controlled family study. *American Journal of Psychiatry, 144,* 330–333.

Biederman, J., Munir, K., Knee, D., Habelow, W., Armentano, M., Autor, S., Hoge, S. K., & Waternaux, C. (1986). A family study of patients with attention deficit disorder and normal controls. *Journal of Psychiatric Research, 20,* 263–274.

Biederman, J., Newcorn, J., & Sprich, S. (1991). Comorbidity of attention deficit hyperactivity disorder with conduct, depressive, anxiety, and other disorders. *American Journal of Psychiatry, 148,* 564–577.

Bird, H. R., Canino, G., Rubio-Stipec, M., Gould, M. S., Ribera, J., Sesman, M., Woodbury, M., Huertas-Goldman, S., Pagan, A., Sanchez-Lacay, A., & Moscoso, M. (1988). Estimates of the prevalence of childhood maladjustment in a community survey in Puerto Rico. *Archives of General Psychiatry, 45,* 1120–1126.

Breslau, N., Davis, G. C., & Prabucki, K. (1988). Depressed mothers as informants in family history research—Are they accurate? *Psychiatry Research, 24,* 345–359.

Carlson, G. A., & Cantwell, D. P. (1980). Unmasking masked depression in children and adolescents. *American Journal of Psychiatry, 137,* 445–449.

Cohen, P., Cohen, J., & Brook, J. (1993). An epidemiological study of disorders in late childhood and adolescence: II. Persistence of disorders. *Journal of Child Psychology and Psychiatry, 34,* 869–877.

Gittelman, R., Mannuzza, S., Shenker, R., & Bonagura, N. (1985). Hyperactive boys almost grown-up: I. Psychiatric status. *Archives of General Psychiatry, 42,* 937–947.

Hammen, C. (1991). *Depression runs in families.* New York: Springer-Verlag.

Keller, M. B., Beardslee, W., Lavori, P. W., Wunder, J., Samuelson, D. L., & Samuelson, H. (1988). Course of major depression in non-referred adolescents: A retrospective study. *Journal of Affective Disorders, 15,* 235–243.

Klein, R. G., & Mannuzza, S. (1990, October). *Psychiatric family history in ADHD.* Paper presented at the annual meeting of the American Academy of Child and Adolescent Psychiatry, Chicago.

Klein, R. G., & Mannuzza, S. (1991). Long-term outcome of hyperactive children: A review. *Journal of the American Academy of Child and Adolescent Psychiatry, 30,* 383–387.

Lahey, B. B., Piacentini, J. C., McBurnett, K., Stone, P., Hartdagen, S., & Hynd, G. (1988). Psychopathology in the parents of children with conduct disorder and hyperactivity. *Journal of the American Academy of Child and Adolescent Psychiatry, 27,* 163–170.

Lewinsohn, P. M., Hops, H., Roberts, R. E., Seeley, J. R., & Andrews, J. A. (1993). Adolescent psychopathology: I. Prevalence and incidence of depression and other DSM-III-R disorders in high school students. *Journal of Abnormal Psychology, 102,* 133–144.

Mannuzza, S., Klein, R. G., Bessler, A., Malloy, P., & LaPadula, M. (1993). Adult outcome of hyperactive boys: I. Educational achievement, occupational rank, and psychiatric status. *Archives of General Psychiatry, 50,* 565–576.

Mannuzza, S., Klein, R. G., Bonagura, N., Malloy, P., Giampino, T. L., & Addalli, K. A. (1991). Hyperactive boys almost grown up: V. Replication of psychiatric status. *Archives of General Psychiatry, 48,* 77–83.

McClellan, J. M., Rubert, M. P., Reichler, R. J., & Sylvester, C. E. (1990). Attention deficit disorder in children at risk for anxiety and depression. *Journal of the American Academy of Child and Adolescent Psychiatry, 29,* 534–539.

Orvaschel, H., Walsh-Allis, G., & Ye, W. (1988). Psychopathology in children of parents with recurrent depression. *Journal of Abnormal Child Psychology, 16,* 17–28.

Puig-Antich, J. (1982). Major depression and conduct disorder in prepuberty. *Journal of the American Academy of Child Psychiatry, 21,* 118–128.

Puig-Antich, J., & Gittelman, R. (1982). Depression in childhood and adolescence. In E. S. Paykel (Ed.), *Handbook of affective disorders* (pp. 379–392). London: Churchill Livingstone.

Schachar, R., & Wachsmuth, R. (1990). Hyperactivity and parental psychopathology. *Journal of Child Psychology and Psychiatry, 31,* 381–392.

Staton, R. D., & Brumback, R. A. (1981). Non-specificity of motor hyperactivity as a diagnostic criterion. *Preceptual and Motor Skills, 52,* 323–332.

Stewart, M. A., & Morrison, J. R. (1973). Affective disorders among the relatives of hyperactive children. *Journal of Child Psychology and Psychiatry, 14,* 209–212.

CHAPTER 16

Chronic Depression in Childhood

Maria Kovacs

The definition and nosological status of dysthymic disorder (DD) has been controversial ever since it was designated in DSM-III (American Psychiatric Association, 1980) as a form of affective disorder (Akiskal, 1983). For example, questions have been raised about its diagnostic validity and whether it is symptomatically distinct from major depressive disorder (MDD) (Howland & Thase, 1991; Kocsis & Frances, 1987). However, the current nosological controversy is not surprising. Indeed, it is only the latest chapter in a long ongoing debate as to whether chronic depression is a form of neuroticism or character pathology, an attenuated or milder version of depressive illness, or a sequela of MDD (Akiskal, 1983, 1989, 1991; Cassano et al., 1983; Kocsis & Frances, 1987). Recently, the controversy has been rekindled by data suggesting that in clinical samples of adult dysthymics, up to 95% have a superimposed MDD (Akiskal, 1983; Kocsis et al., 1986), and among those with MDD, as many as one-third have an underlying DD (Alnaes & Torgersen, 1989; Keller et al., 1982). That is, the identification of "double depression" (MDD superimposed upon DD) has raised additional questions about whether DD should be diagnosed as a disorder separate from MDD (Keller & Lavori, 1984).

Chronic depression that has its onset in childhood or adolescence has long been regarded as one of the prototypical forms of this condition. There appear to be at least two subtypes of such early onset chronic depressions; one is a form of bona fide affective disorder ("subaffective dysthymia") and the other is "characterological" in nature (Akiskal, 1991; Akiskal et al., 1980). In DSM-III-R (American Psychiatric Association, 1987), the importance of early onset also is acknowledged. DD is described as typically beginning in childhood or adolescence, with attention-deficit disorder, conduct disorder, and "severe" specific developmental disorders as putative risk factors and psychoactive substance abuse as one of its eventual complications.

However, until recently, the existence of early onset chronic depression was supported primarily by retrospective reports of adult patients. In fact, the Pittsburgh longitudinal study of childhood onset depressive disorders, started in 1978, generated the earliest reports on dysthymia in childhood and its frequent comorbidity with major depression (Kovacs et al., 1984a, 1984b). Since then, other investigators have confirmed in clinical, nonclinical, and epidemiological samples of youths the existence of DD and its cooccurrence with MDD (Anderson et al., 1987; Mitchell et al., 1988; Kashani et al., 1987; Keller et al., 1988). Dysthymia in very young patients allows a direct examination of the disorder in its bona fide, early onset form. Therefore, questions that have been posed about its relationship to MDD may be more readily explored in juvenile cohorts, including the extent to which the two conditions are symptomatically distinct. In addition, the longitudinal study of children with DD can resolve questions about the predictive validity of the diagnoses. If childhood onset dysthymia is a form of affective disorder, the likelihood of affective disorder later in adolescence and young adulthood should exceed the likelihood of other outcomes.

The purpose of this chapter is to review findings from the Pittsburgh prospective longitudinal study concerning the characteristics and diagnostic validity of DD in childhood, diagnosed according to DSM-III. The initial presentation, pattern of recovery, and subsequent course and outcome of dysthymia are described, including the sequence and rates of the various types of secondary disorders and symptom-free periods over an up to 12-year interval of study observation. To enable readers to judge the generalizability and the clinical implications of the findings, a brief overview of the study design is presented first.

Design of the Pittsburgh Longitudinal Study

As described elsewhere (Kovacs et al., 1984a), subjects for the Pittsburgh longitudinal study were recruited over a period of several years, with the child psychiatry clinic of the University of Pittsburgh (Pennsylvania) contributing the vast majority of cases; suitability for the study was determined by the research staff. Children had to meet a set of demographic study inclusionary criteria, including age of 8 to 13 years, no mental retardation, no major systemic medical illness, ambulatory psychiatric and medical status, and living with parent(s) or legal guardian(s) and within commuting distance of Greater Pittsburgh. Written consents were obtained for an initial 5-year follow-up period and then for optional further follow-up periods. The protocol stipulated three postintake assessments in the first year of study participation and no more than two interviews every year thereafter.

To minimize information variance, clinical evaluations were conducted with the semistructured, symptom-oriented Interview Schedule for Children (intake and follow-up versions) and its addenda (Kovacs, 1985). At each clinical assessment, first the parent was interviewed alone about the child, then the child was interviewed separately by the same clinician. Structured data sheets also were used with the parents to gather anamnestic, demographic, and other interim information at each contact. Subsequent to each interview, the subject's psychiatric diagnosis was based on the clinician's final symptom ratings, taking into account pertinent historical information. Only symptoms at operationally predefined levels of severity counted toward a diagnosis. The repeated assessments were reviewed by the clinicians, and final diagnoses were consensually assigned, using the DSM-III criteria, but hierarchical diagnostic rules were not always applied.

The approach to diagnosing concurrent disorders that had overlapping and similar symptoms has been illustrated in several articles (Kovacs et al., 1984a, 1984b). With regard to an episode of MDD superimposed upon a long-standing dysthymia, there were two common presentations. The dysthymic child showed new symptoms by virtue of which he or she also met criteria for MDD (e.g., in addition to the preexisting dysthymic picture, the child developed appetite disturbance and fatigue). In the alternate presentation, a dysthymic symptom changed sufficiently (e.g., inability to respond with pleasure to praise merged into clear-cut anhedonia) and/or previous subclinical symptoms exacerbated to criterion levels such that the child qualified for the additional diagnosis of MDD. Thus, in the case of double depression, some symptoms were counted toward both diagnoses. Even if the chronic minor affective disturbance appeared to be prodromal to MDD, if the former met DSM-III criteria for DD, it was so diagnosed; on the other hand, a partially remitted MDD (even if chronic) was not diagnosed as DD. Parents were the primary informants for chronological data, and both the onset of a disorder and offset, or recovery, were operationally defined (Kovacs et al., 1984a, 1984b, in press).

The Sample and Follow-Up Interval

The depressed cohort of the Pittsburgh longitudinal study ($n = 142$) consists of several subgroups defined by their index (study entry) diagnosis, three of which are pertinent to this chapter, namely: children with MDD but no history of DD ($n = 60$), children with DD ($n = 23$), and children with both an MDD and an underlying DD ($n = 32$). There is also a psychiatric control group with miscellaneous diagnoses but no current or past depression ($n = 49$). The subjects of this chapter are the children with a diagnosis of DD at study entry. The nondysthymic, or "pure" MDD, and the control cases are used for some comparisons.

Of the 55 dysthymic children, 28 were girls (51%) and most children were white (69%). Their ages ranged from 8.0 to 13.9 (mean = 11.14 years) at study entry. Socioeconomic status (SES), according to Hollingshead's (1957) two-factor index, indicated an overrepresentation of lower SES (categories IV, V; 71%). Children with DD ($n = 55$) and those with MDD ($n = 60$) were similar in both gender distribution and mean age at study entry, whereas the nondepressed comparison cases were mostly boys ($p = .002$) and about 7 to 10 months younger on average ($p = .03$). The dysthymics did not differ from the major depressive and control groups in SES, dichotomized into high (I, II, III) versus low (IV, V) ($p = .17$).

At study entry, only 14 dysthymic children (25.5%) were living in intact families, and altogether 30 (54.5%) were living in two-parent households. Four children (7.3%) had a history of inpatient psychiatric hospitalization, 20 (36.4%) had past outpatient psychosocial treatment, and 5 (9.1%) had received psychotropic medications in the past. There were no significant differences between the DD, MDD, and control groups on any of the foregoing variables (p's between .13 and .87).

The data summarized in this chapter were restricted to information collected up to September 1, 1990 ("criterion interview"). This corresponded to a follow-up period of a maximum of 12.1 years (minimum of 3 years), with a mean of 6.4 years for nondropouts, and an average follow-up period of 0.7 year (range = 0.1 to 1.7 years) for nine DD cases who dropped out/were lost. At the criterion interview, mean age was 17.7 years, with a range from 12.5 years to 23.7 years.

Initial Presentation of Dysthymia

One of the notable features of the dysthymic children in the present study is that they represent an entirely first-episode cohort. The age at onset of DD among these children ranged from 5.2 to 12.8 years (mean = 8.7 years). Compared to the group of children whose first affective episode was major depression, it was found that first-episode DD had a significantly earlier onset than first-episode MDD (8.7 vs. 10.9 years). When they entered the study, 32 children (58.2%) already had a superimposed episode of MDD, or double depression, and six others developed an MDD later on during their DD. Thus, altogether 69.1% of the children had at least one episode of MDD *superimposed* upon their DD disorder.

In addition, as described in detail elsewhere (Kovacs et al., 1994), only about 53% of the cases had primary dysthymia. Among the rest of the children, the pre-existing conditions clearly predated the onset of the DD and were still present at the time the DD started. Attention-deficit disorder was the most prevalent preexisting disorder (23.6%), followed by enuresis/encopresis (14.6%). Various types of anxiety disorders accounted for about 22% of the preexisting conditions. In comparison, 62% of the index MDD group had preexisting disorders, with 17% having had attention-deficit disorder. One of the controversies regarding DD has been whether its symptomatic presentation is distinct from that of MDD. As one approach to this dilemma, children with a full-blown DD (but no MDD) and children in a full-blown episode of MDD (but no concurrent dysthymia) were compared in the frequencies of selected symptoms. The Pittsburgh data indicate that dysthymia in childhood is predominantly characterized by persistently gloomy and depressed mood (92% of the cases) and brooding (typically about feeling unloved) and additional symptoms of affective dysregulation, including irritability (56%) and anger (64%). The other noted feature is the "cognitive" symptom of self-deprecation (56%). At the same time, childhood dysthymia (as compared to MDD) is notable for the almost virtual absence of anhedonia (5.6%) and social withdrawal (8.3%), the comparatively low rates of guilt, morbid preoccupation, and impaired concentration (14% to 42%), the virtual absence of reduced appetite (5.6%), and the low rates of hyposomnia (22%) and fatigue (22%).

Recovery from the First Episode of Dysthymia

Preliminary data on a portion of the sample had already suggested that although childhood onset dysthymia is associated with a high rate of eventual recovery, the episode is protracted (Kovacs et al., 1984a). These early indications were recently reconfirmed by examining all the cases after they were observed sufficiently long for them to have recovered. As reported elsewhere (Kovacs et al., in press), first-episode dysthymia is indeed protracted. The average episode length for recovered cases is close to 4 years. Plotting the rate of recovery cumulatively reveals that the likelihood of remission is gradual; after the first year of illness (required in DSM-III to meet diagnostic criteria), no particular 6-month period is associated with a high likelihood of recovery. However, eventually, 98% of the children recover from their first episodes, although it takes up to 8 years from onset to reach that proportion of cumulative recovery.

Preliminary data on a portion of the cohort revealed that having a superimposed MDD or an anxiety disorder along the course of DD did not affect the likelihood of recovery but age at onset did; those who were younger took somewhat longer to recover (Kovacs et al., 1984a). In examining the entire sample after most of them have recovered, the findings about superimposed depression were confirmed. In addition, using a multivariate modeling procedure, having a preexisting conduct/attention-deficit disorder was found to lengthen the episode by about 2 years on average. After that was taken into consideration, age at onset was no longer significant in explaining the rate of recovery.

Diagnostic Course of Dysthymia

One way to describe course and outcome is to examine the kind of disorders that develop secondary to DD onset. As noted elsewhere, an episode of major depression was the most frequent complication; altogether, 42 cases experienced it (Kovacs et al., 1994). In addition, seven dysthymics developed Bipolar I or II disorders. However, a "direct" switch from DD to bipolarity was infrequent; the more typical course was dysthymia leading to major depression, eventually culminating in bipolar illness. All in all, only one-fifth of the sample did *not* develop some form of affective disorder over the follow-up. And, contrary to DSM-III-R, substance use/abuse disorders were relatively infrequent complications of DD (7.3%). These findings were reconfirmed by using survival analysis and life-table methods (Kalbfleisch & Prentice, 1980), which take into account that observation periods vary across cases and yield estimates of the survival (time-to-response) distribution for the entire cohort. With time, MDD was found to be the outcome of greatest likelihood. The maximum cumulative probability of .81 for the first episode of MDD is reached by 8.5 years after DD onset. The highest-risk period was the second to third year of DD. Bipolar illness developing, with a cumulative probability of .21, also represents a notable outcome, whereas cumulative risk (.11) of substance use disorder secondary to DD is low.

The chronological sequence of major psychiatric disorders that developed secondary to DD was also examined, up to the fifth new secondary disorder. "V" codes, adjustment disorders, enuresis/encopresis, and recurrent episodes of a disorder were not tallied. Consistent with the previously presented data, almost all the children (91%, $n = 50$) developed at least one, and most children (73%, $n = 40$) developed two new disorders subsequent to the onset of their dysthymia. Among those with at least one new condition, MDD was the most frequent and an anxiety disorder the next most frequent. Among the children who developed two conditions, the most likely diagnoses were MDD, separation anxiety disorder, and conduct disorder. Taking into account all the conditions that emerged, affective disorders still remained the outcomes of greatest likelihood.

Furthermore, a schematic presentation of the actual sequencing of all affective disorder outcomes (up to the criterion interview) in the dysthymic sample and among the index MDD cases revealed two notable findings. First, it appeared that, after DD onset, a first episode of MDD was the "gateway" for all (except two) subsequent affective disorder episodes. That is, *after* developing the first episode of MDD, the dysthymic child is at risk for a second episode of MDD (38%), a first episode of bipolar illness (13%), a second episode of DD (9%), and a first episode of cyclothymia (2%), roughly in that order of likelihood. Second, when the starting point is the first episode of MDD, the sequence of affective disorders for the index DD and the index MDD groups appear to be comparable. That is, approximately one-third of the children with a first episode of MDD develop a second MDD episode, and about 15% develop bipolar illness.

Given that close to 50% of the sample had a disorder prior to their DD, and that 91% developed at least one diagnosable condition subsequently, the question arises as to whether such youths are chronically ill. In order to answer this question, the data were examined for symptom-free periods. As the years pass, children with DD were found to be "well," or free of diagnosable psychiatric illness only about one-third of the time on average. Their symptomatic or "ill" periods are accounted for by a variety of disorders, including depression. However, the fact that they are "free" of affective disorder close to 50% of the time underscores the episodic nature of these conditions on long-term follow-up.

Research and Clinical Significance

Childhood onset DD, diagnosed according to the DSM-III, is a form of affective illness, as reflected by its longitudinal course and outcome, notwithstanding the fact that it may present either as a primary or secondary disorder. Therefore, the findings of the Pittsburgh longitudinal study reconfirm and extend the work and theoretical formulations of Akiskal (1983, 1991) on adults, as well as recent empirical observations by others. Specifically, the dysthymic children in the present sample represented an entirely first-episode cohort, without any prior known history of major depression. They had a mean age of onset of 8.7 years, 52% had primary dysthymia, and an eventual superimposed episode of MDD was common (69% of the sample). DD appears to be symptomatically distinct from MDD and is notable for the relative absence of anhedonia, guilt, and certain neurovegetative disturbances. Furthermore, the clinical course of childhood onset DD is characterized by recovery followed by subsequent "affective" episodes and sporadic symptom-free intervals.

As suggested by DSM-III-R, attention-deficit disorder (ADD) was a frequent preexisting condition in the present sample. However, it is not clear whether ADD is a specific risk factor, partly because cases were not selected based on presence or absence of ADD and partly because its putative "risk" value depends on its base rate in clinically referred samples. In any case, the rates of preexisting or comorbid nonaffective disorders do not appear to differentiate childhood onset MDD and DD. However, the age-of-onset dimension appears to hold some promise for differentiating childhood onset DD and MDD, given that first-episode DD appears to have an earlier onset than first-episode MDD. In the present study, children were 8.7 years, on average, at the onset of their dysthymia. They tended to be about 11.4 years old when they developed a first MDD, which is similar to the mean age of onset of MDD of 10.9 years in the nondysthymic sample. Lewinsohn et al. (1991), in their community sample of adolescents, also reported an earlier onset of first depressive episode for DD cases as compared to MDD cases.

Although dysthymia is protracted, the probability of recovery is high. And, as far as the first episode is concerned, it does not persist into adulthood. The mean length of the index episode is about 4 years, and recovery is gradual. These data strongly suggest that childhood onset DD is a serious disorder that can be expected to affect young patients' functioning because they remain symptomatic for a long time. With regard to the symptomatology of DD, several comments are in order. First, in clinical samples of adults, the difficulty of locating "pure" dysthymics (e.g., Akiskal, 1983; Keller & Sessa, 1990) has precluded a comparison of DD and MDD symptoms. On the other hand, in an epidemiological cohort of adults, Angst and Wicki (1991) could not symptomatically distinguish the two diagnostic groups. However, at least in childhood, DD may be clinically distinguished from an episode of MDD, and is characterized predominantly by dysphoric mood and additional signs of affective dysregulation: There is an absence of anhedonia and certain neurovegetative symptoms. Social withdrawal is also relatively rare. Although Fine et al. (1985) could not distinguish these disorders in their study of clinically referred youths, they had very small samples, and their comparisons were made using mean symptom ratings, as opposed to the strategy employed in the Pittsburgh study.

Childhood onset dysthymia is a form of affective illness, characterized by recurrences and well periods, as opposed to its being a characterological or "trait-like" condition. It is also a risk factor for eventual bipolarity. Although the base rate of bipolar illness in clinical samples of children and youths has not been firmly established, the cumulative risk of .21 is clearly notable and worrisome. This finding was unexpected. However, the association between DD and bipolar illness among adults has been described by Akiskal (1983; Akiskal et al., 1983; Rosenthal et al., 1981) and was subsequently reconfirmed by Klein et al. (1988) and others as well (Rihmer, 1990; Wicki & Angst, 1991). Furthermore, it is notable that in one series of depressed patients examined by Akiskal et al. (1983), switching from unipolar to bipolar illness (most common in young adulthood) characterized 20% of the sample, and most of those who switched had early onset illness. Indeed, Akiskal et al. (1989) recently proposed that both episodic and chronic depressions, including bipolar I and II forms, be viewed as components of a broad affective spectrum.

In the literature on adults, one of the questions has been whether MDD, DD, and their co-occurring forms are distinct nosological entities or merely phases of the same disorder, or specifically, whether there is utility to recognizing double depression (Keller & Lavori, 1984). Empiric attempts to answer these questions have focused on whether patients with double depression can be distinguished from those with pure recurrent MDD on clinical, functional, and historic variables. The results have been equivocal (e.g., Klein et al., 1988; Kocsis et al., 1986; Miller et al., 1986). The situation appears to be somewhat different among children and adolescents. Although the vast majority of childhood dysthymics develop superimposed major depression, and their *subsequent* naturalistic course may not be distinguishable from those youths whose first illness is MDD, dysthymia is symptomatically distinct and should be separately identified. In addition, there is at least a 2-year-long period before the first superimposed episode of MDD occurs. Therefore, in juvenile cohorts with DD, there may be an unparalleled opportunity to explore the value of early identification and prevention of recurrent episodes of affective illness.

Finally, it should be noted that in the present, first-episode cohort, dysthymia was *not* a residual condition. Chronic sequelae or residual states of affective disorders among adults have been long recognized (e.g., Cassano et al., 1983; Keller & Sessa, 1990), with approximately 15% to 20% of adult MDD patients having such outcomes. Therefore, one unresolved issue concerns the similarities or differences among DD children and those with chronic, partially remitted MDD. Furthermore, the generalizability of the findings of the Pittsburgh study to nonreferred and/or untreated populations is, as of now, not known. A related concern is that subsequent to the intake evaluations and the cases' initial diagnostic assignment, the follow-up assessments were not blind to the results of prior research interviews. Therefore, some degree of diagnostic bias cannot be entirely ruled out. Another research issue concerns diagnostic validators of childhood onset DD other than clinical course. Several indexes of diagnostic validity that have shown promise in the study of adults, including tricyclic antidepressant response and biological markers, such as rapid eye movement latency, do not appear to be useful in the preadult years. Establishing definite family history of psychiatric illness on the paternal side can also be problematic because of the high rate of early divorces and never-married parents, resulting in partial or no information about many fathers in clinically referred samples. Therefore, alternative ways of establishing diagnostic validity for childhood onset DD also remain a research priority. To date, prospective follow-up represents the most robust validating strategy. As illustrated in this chapter, such follow-up tends to establish dysthymia as a mood disorder with protracted phases, each phase extending over an average of 4 years. In adults, these phases seem to coalesce into a more chronic indefinite course with remissions that do not generally exceed weeks at a time (Akiskal, 1983)—hence, developing clinical interventions for dysthymic children may have great public health significance.

Acknowledgments

This work was supported by Grant MH-33990 from the National Institute of Mental Health, Health and Human Services Administration, Bethesda, Maryland, and by a grant from the W. T. Grant Foundation, New York, New York. Particular appreciation is expressed to Phoebe Lucy Parrone for conducting computer programming tasks.

References

Akiskal, H. S. (1983). Dysthymic disorder: Psychopathology of proposed chronic depressive subtypes. *American Journal of Psychiatry, 140,* 11–20.

Akiskal, H. S. (1989). New insights into the nature and heterogeneity of mood disorders. *Journal of Clinical Psychiatry, 50*(Suppl.), 6–12.

Akiskal, H. S. (1991). Chronic depression. *Bulletin of the Menninger Clinic, 55,* 156–171.

Akiskal, H. S., Cassano, G. B., Musetti, L., Perugi, G., Tundo, A., & Mignani, V. (1989). Psychopathology, temperament, and past course in primary major depressions. 1. Review of evidence for a bipolar spectrum. *Psychopathology, 22,* 268–277.

Akiskal, H. S., Rosenthal, T. L., Haykal, R. F., Lemmi, H., Rosenthal, R. H., & Scott-Strauss, A. (1980). Characterological depressions. *Archives of General Psychiatry, 37,* 777–783.

Akiskal, H. S., Walker, P., Puzantian, V. R., King, D., Rosenthal, T. L., & Dranon, M. (1983). Bipolar outcome in the course of depressive illness: Phenomenologic, familial, and pharmacologic predictors. *Journal of Affective Disorders, 5,* 115–128.

Alnaes, R., & Torgersen, S. (1989). Characteristics of patients with major depression in combination with dysthymic or cyclothymic disorders. *Acta Psychiatrica Scandinavica, 79,* 11–18.

American Psychiatric Association. (1980). *Diagnostic and statistical manual of mental disorders* (3rd ed.). Washington, DC: Author.

American Psychiatric Association. (1987). *Diagnostic and statistical manual of mental disorders* (3rd ed., rev.). Washington, DC: Author.

Anderson, J. C., Williams, S., McGee, R., & Silva, P. A. (1987). DSM-III disorders in preadolescent children: Prevalence in a large sample from the general population. *Archives of General Psychiatry, 44,* 69–76.

Angst, J., & Wicki, W. (1991). The Zurich study: XI. Is dysthymia a separate form of depression? Results of the Zurich cohort study. *European Archives of Psychiatry and Clinical Neuroscience, 240,* 349–354.

Cassano, G. B., Maggini, C., & Akiskal, H. S. (1983). Short-term, subchronic, and chronic sequelae of affective disorders. *Psychiatric Clinics of North America, 6,* 55–67.

Fine, S., Moretti, M., Haley, G., & Marriage, K. (1985). Affective disorders in children and adolescents: The dysthymic disorder dilemma. *Canadian Journal of Psychiatry, 30,* 173–177.

Hollingshead, A. B. (1957). *Two Factor Index of Social Position.* New Haven, CT: Yale University Sociology Department.

Howland, R. H., & Thase, M. E. (1991). Biological studies of dysthymia. *Biological Psychiatry, 30,* 283–304.

Kalbfleisch, J. D., & Prentice, R. L. (1980). *The statistical analysis of failure time data.* New York: Wiley.

Kashani, J. H., Carlson, G. A., Beck, N. C., Hoeper, E. W., Corcoran, C. M., McAllister, J. A., Fallani, C., Rosenberg, T. K., & Reid, J. C. (1987). Depression, depressive symptoms, and depressed mood among a community sample of adolescents. *American Journal of Psychiatry, 144,* 931–934.

Keller, M. B., Beardslee, W., Lavori, P. W., Wunder, J., Ors, D. L., & Samuelson, H. (1988). Course of major depression in nonreferred adolescents: A retrospective study. *Journal of Affective Disorders, 15,* 235–243.

Keller, M. B., & Lavori, P. W. (1984). Double depression, major depression, and dysthymia: Distinct entities or different phases of a single disorder? *Psychopharmacology Bulletin, 20,* 399–402.

Keller, M. B., & Sessa, F. M. (1990). Dysthymia: Development and clinical course. In S. Burton & H. Akiskal (Eds.), *Dysthymic disorder* (pp. 13–23). London: Gaskell.

Keller, M. B., Shapiro, R. W., Lavori, P. W., & Wolfe, N. (1982). Recovery in major depressive disorder: Analysis with the life table and regression models. *Archives of General Psychiatry, 39,* 905–910.

Klein, D. N., Taylor, E. B., Harding, K., & Dickstein, S. (1988). Double depression and episodic major depression: Demographic, clinical, familial, personality, and socioenvironmental characteristics and short-term outcome. *American Journal of Psychiatry, 145,* 1226–1231.

Kocsis, J. H., & Frances, A. J. (1987). A critical discussion of DSM-III dysthymic disorder. *American Journal of Psychiatry, 144,* 1534–1542.

Kocsis, J. H., Voss, C., Mann, J. J., & Francis, A. (1986). Chronic depression: Demographic and clinical characteristics. *Psychopharmacology Bulletin, 22,* 192–195.

Kovacs, M. (1985). The Interview Schedule for Children (ISC). *Psychopharmacology Bulletin, 21,* 991–994.

Kovacs, M., Akiskal, H. S., Gatsonis, C., & Parrone, P. L. (1994). Childhood-onset dysthymic disorder: Clinical features and prospective naturalistic outcome. *Archives of General Psychiatry, 51,* 365–374.

Kovacs, M., Feinberg, T. L., Crouse-Novak, M. A., Paulauskas, S. L., & Finkelstein, R. (1984a). Depressive disorders in childhood: I. A longitudinal prospective study of characteristics and recovery. *Archives of General Psychiatry, 41,* 229–237.

Kovacs, M., Feinberg, T. L., Crouse-Novak, M., Paulauskas, S. L., Pollock, M., & Finkelstein, R. (1984b). Depressive disorders in childhood: II. A longitudinal study of the risk for a subsequent major depression. *Archives of General Psychiatry, 41,* 643–649.

Kovacs, M., Gatsonis, C., Obrosky, D. S., & Richards, C. (in press). First episode major depressive and dysthymic disorders in childhood: Clinical and sociodemographic factors in recovery. *Journal of the American Academy of Child and Adolescent Psychiatry.*

Lewinsohn, P. M., Rohde, P., Seeley, J. R., & Hops, H. (1991). Comorbidity of unipolar depression: I. Major depression with dysthymia. *Journal of Abnormal Psychology, 100,* 205–213.

Miller, I. W., Norman, W. H., & Dow, M. G. (1986). Psychosocial characteristics of "double depression." *American Journal of Psychiatry, 143,* 1042–1044.

Mitchell, J., McCauley, E., Burke, P. M., & Moss, S. J. (1988). Phenomenology of depression in children and adolescents. *Journal of the American Academy of Child and Adolescent Psychiatry, 27,* 12–20.

Rihmer, Z. (1990). Dysthymia: A clinician's perspective. In S. Burton & H. Akiskal (Eds.), *Dysthymic disorder* (pp. 112–125). London: Gaskell.

Rosenthal, T. L., Akiskal, H. S., Scott-Strauss, A., Rosenthal, R. H., & David, M. (1981). Bipolar outcome in the course of depressive illness: Phenomenologic, familial, and pharmacologic predictors. *Journal of Affective Disorders, 3,* 183–192.

Wicki, W., & Angst, J. (1991). The Zurich study: X. Hypomania in a 28- to 30-year old cohort. *European Archives of Psychiatry and Clinical Neuroscience, 240,* 339–348.

Index

ACTH response to CRH, 154
Acute treatment, desipramine, 69–71
Adjustment reactions, 5
Adrenal insufficiency, 154
Affective dysregulation (*see* Mood disorders)
Age of onset
  and drug response, 46–51
  dysthymic children, 211, 215
    and recovery, 213
  minor depression, 188
  neurotic depression, 116, 117
  recurrent brief depression, 188
Alcoholism
  dysthymia comorbidity, 37, 38
  family history, 50, 141, 142
  and residual depression, 16
Amisulpride, 20, 27
Amitriptyline
  anger cause, 178
  fibromyalgia treatment, 155
  long-term study, 40
  neurotic depression response, 118
Anger, and imipramine, 178
Angry depression
  in children, 212
  neurotic depression relationship, 114, 115
Anhedonia
  childhood dysthymia, absence of, 212, 215
  in DSM definitions, 139
Antidepressants
  chronic dysphoria response, 174–180
  dysthymia response, 14, 15
  dysthymia subgroups response, 46–51
Antisocial personality traits, 49

Anxiety states
  chronic depression profile, 61
  drug response, 49, 50, 71
  neurotic depression demarcation, 109–112
  tense arousal in, 150
Anxious depression, 5, 6
Arousal, 150
Attention-deficit/hyperactivity disorder, 198–205
  age of onset, 199
  clinical studies, 199, 200
  and dysthymia, 198–205, 212, 215
  family studies, 200–203
  gender differences, 199
  in girls, 203, 204
  longitudinal studies, 203, 204
  major depression association, 198–205
Atypical depression, 165–171
  clinical heterogeneity, 3–10
  comorbidity, 56
  endogenous depression overlap, 169–171
  grade of membership analysis, 170
  history, 165
  meaning of, 3, 4, 165, 166
  monoamine oxidase inhibitor response, 165–169
  symptomatology, 7, 8
Axis II disorders (*see* Personality disorders)

B

Back pain, 169
Beck Depression Inventory, 61, 67
Behavior-disordered children, 199, 200
Bipolar diathesis, 21, 22

Bipolar disorder
  and attention-deficit/hyperactivity disor-
    der, 205
  childhood dysthymia outcome, 213, 215,
    216
  chronicity, 57, 58
  depressive personality association, 92
  negative social consequences, 81, 82
  neurotic depression difference, 120, 121
  residual states, 75–84
  unipolar disorder biological kinship, 120
Bipolar II depression
  anxiety states, 6
  atypical symptomatology, 4
  chronicity, 57, 58
Borderline personality disorder
  chronic dyphorias relationship, 178, 179
  and depressive personality, 91
  drug response, 178, 179
  labeling effects, and treatment failure, 22
Borg Scale, 149
Brief recurrent depression (*see* Recurrent
  brief depression)

C

Carbamazepine, 17
Categorical classifications, 112, 113, 119,
  132
Characterological depression
  classification, 45
  clinical features, 8, 9
  drug treatment response, 46–51
  family studies, 9
  fluoxetine response, 21
  pharmacological dissection, 18, 19, 46–
    51
Children, 208–217
  attention-deficit/hyperactivity disorder,
    198–205, 212, 215
  double depression, 216
  dysthymia, 208–217
    family studies, 13
  Pittsburgh longitudinal study, 209–217
China, neurasthenia diagnosis, 6, 156
Chocolate craving, 8
Chronic dysphorias, 174–180
Chronic fatigue syndrome, 148–159
  differential diagnosis, 155–158
  and neurasthenia, 6, 7, 148, 149
  working case definition, 151, 152
Chronic mononucleosis, 151
Chronic pain, 169

Clinical Global Evaluation of Improvement, 46, 47
Cluster analysis
  limitations, 78, 79
  neurotic-endogenous depression, 119,
    132, 133
Cognitive psychotherapy, 122
"Combined depression," 195
Comorbidity
  atypical depression, 56
  chronicity link, 56
  desipramine response, 71
  neurotic depression, 107, 108
  primary dysthymia, 37, 38
Conduct disorder, 200, 201
Continuation treatment, desipramine, 69
Continuum concept
  Kraepelin's view, 97, 98
  neurotic-endogenous depression, 112,
    113, 119
  and pharmacological dissection, 19
Cornell Dysthymia Rating Scale, 67
Countertransference, 25
Cytokines, 153

D

Demoralization, 5
Dependent–histrionic personality
  drug treatment response, 49
  monoamine oxidase inhibitors in, 20
La dépression constitutionelle, 12
Depression-prone personality, 12
Depression spectrum disease, 19
Depressive disorder not otherwise speci-
  fied, 138–141
Depressive personality, 87–94
  college student sample, 91–93
  criteria, 88, 89
  DSM classification, 87, 88, 94
  dysthymia relationship, 12, 87–94
  family history, 90, 93
  and major depression, 87, 94
  mood disorders association, 89, 90
  and schizotypal personality, 90
Depressive temperament (*see* Tempera-
  ment)
Desipramine, 18, 68–71
"Dichotomous" view, 112, 113, 119, 132
Disability Assessment Schedule, 78, 81,
  82
Discontinuation studies, desipramine, 69
Divalproex augmentation, 22

"Double depression"
  in children, 216
  as classification artifact, 67
  clinical presentation, 13
  community sample, 36
  drug response, 177
  suicide attempts, 196
Drug response (*see also* Pharmacological
    dissection)
  chronic dysphoria, 175–189
  definition, 67
  neurotic depression, 118, 177
  nosological implications, 122
  unipolar and bipolar disorders, 120
Drug use/abuse, 213
DSM-II, neurotic depression, 96
DSM-III
  depressive personality, 87, 88
  dysthymia, 10, 87, 88, 103, 137
  European psychiatrists' attitudes, 130, 131
  neurotic depression dismissal, 133, 134,
    136–138
  impact of, 119–123
  replacement categories, 136–138
DSM-III-R
  depressive personality, 87, 88
  dysthymia, 10–12, 87, 88
  neurotic depression replacement catego-
    ries, 138, 139
DSM-IV
  depressive personality, 88, 94
  dysthymia, 10–12, 88
  neurotic depression elimination, impact,
    119–123
  neurotic depression replacement catego-
    ries, 140, 141
Duration of episode
  chronicity predictor, 58, 59
  and residual depression, 60, 61
Dysmorphophobia, 37, 38
Dysthymia (*see also* Primary dysthymia)
  age of onset, children, 211, 213, 215
  and attention-deficit/hyperactivity disor-
    der, 198, 205, 212, 215
  in children, 208–217
  versus chronic major depression, 62
  chronicity criterion, 102, 105, 106
  comorbidity, 37, 38
  depressive personality relationship, 87–94
  drug response, 177
  DSM classification/criteria, 10, 11, 44,
    45, 103, 105, 106
  endogenous features, 14
  familial loading, 13

long-term pharmacotherapy, outcome,
    18–22, 40, 68–71
  neurotic depression comparison, 96–123
  pharmacological dissection, 18–22, 177
  predictive validity, 14, 15
  prevalence, 45, 194
  recovery in children, 212, 213
  and recurrent brief depression, 194
  stressful life events, 106, 107
  as subaffective disorder, 11–15
  symptom-free periods, children, 214
  symptom profile, 13, 14, 38, 39

E

Early-onset dysthymia (*see also* Age of onset)
  and character structure, 18
  depressive personality association, 89, 90
  drug response, 46–51
Effortful processes
  fatigue relationship, 149, 150, 153
  measurement of, 149, 150
  and neurasthenia, 148–150
Electroconvulsive therapy
  in residual depression, 17
  "retarded" melancholia response, 113, 114
"Emotionally unstable character disorder," 8
Emphatic listening
  dysthymia approach, 24
  neurasthenia, 7
Endogenous depression
  atypical depression overlap, 4
  categorical definition, 113, 119
  dysthymia link, 14
  neurotic depression independence, 102,
    104, 112–114, 132
  temperament relationship, 2
  treatment response, 113
Enuresis/encopresis, 212
Episodic depression (*see also* Recurrent
    brief depression)
  fluoxetine open study, 176, 177
  placebo response, 175, 176
Epstein–Barr virus, 151
"Existential depression," 12, 23

F

Factor analysis (*see* Cluster analysis)
Family history
  attention-deficit/hyperactivity disorder,
    200–203

Family history *(continued)*
  characterological depression, 9, 19
  depressive personality, 90
  dysthymia, 13, 179
  minor depression, 186, 187
  neurotic depression, 4, 108, 109, 120,
    121
  and pharmacotherapy response, 19, 20,
    48, 50
  recurrent brief depression, 186, 187
Fatigue
  atypical depression symptom, 7
  medical causes, 150, 151
  and neurasthenia, 148, 149
  tense arousal in, 150
Fibromyalgia
  diagnostic criteria, 154, 155
  differential diagnosis, 155–158
  treatment, 155
Fluoxetine
  chronic dysphoria response, 176, 177, 179
  dysthymia long-term response, 20–22
  interpersonal sensitivity response, 169
  and pharmacological dissection, 20–22,
    176, 177, 179
Full remission, and desipramine, 69–71
Functional psychoses
  negative social consequences, 81, 82
  phenomenological constellations, 81–84
  residual states, 75–84
"Fuzzy set" principle, 170

G

Gender differences
  attention-deficit/hyperactivity disorder,
    199
  drug treatment response, 48
  minor depression, 186
  neurotic depression, personality, 110–112
  recurrent brief depression, 186
General Behavior Inventory, 88, 92
Generalized anxiety disorder
  depression link, 6
  desipramine response, 71
  dysthymia comorbidity, 37, 38
Genetics *(see* Family history)
Gepirone, 169
Girls, attention-deficit/hyperactivity disor-
    der, 203, 204
Global Assessment Scale, 78, 81, 82
Grade of membership analysis, 170
Guilt, childhood dysthymia, 212

H

Hamilton Rating Scale for Anxiety, 46, 47
Hamilton Rating Scale for Depression, 36,
    39, 40, 46, 47, 49, 50, 67
Health services utilization, 45
Heredity *(see* Family history)
Herpes simplex I, 153
Histrionic traits, 49
Hopkins Symptom Checklist–90, 36, 46, 47
Hostile depression *(see* Angry depression)
Hyperthymic temperament, 55, 59
Hypomania
  and minor depression, 187
  recurrent brief depression association, 9,
    187
  and somatization, 157
Hypothyroidism, and fatigue, 151
Hysteroid dysphorias, 174–180
  borderline personality relationship, 178,
    179
  conceptual issues, 174, 175
  neurotic depression relationship, 114,
    115
  pharmacological responsivity, 174–180
  symptomatology, 8

I

ICD–8/ICD–9, 131
ICD–10
  neurotic depression elimination, impact,
    119–123
  neurotic depression replacement catego-
    ries, 139, 140
  severity staging, 139
Imipramine
  anger cause, 178
  chronic dysphoria response, 175, 176
  dysthymia response, 20
  long-term open study, dysthymia, 40
  neurotic depression response, 118
  short-term controlled study, 67, 68
Immune deficiency, 153
Insight-oriented therapies, 24
Interpersonal psychotherapy
  indications, 24
  neurotic depression response, 122
Interpersonal sensitivity *(see* Rejection sen-
    sitivity)
Interrater reliability, neurotic depression,
    133
Iproniazid, 165

Irritable bowel syndrome, 156, 157
Irritability, childhood dysthymia, 212
Isocarboxazid, 166–168

J

James, William, neurasthenia description,
148

K

Kindling, 100
Kraepelin's theories
bipolar–unipolar disorder unity, 120
and brief recurrent depressions, 9, 10
depressive spectrum, 97, 98
temperament, 2

L

Late-onset dysthymia, 46–51
Length of episode (see Duration of episode)
Lewis's unitary concept, 119
Libido increase, 167
Life-chart course, 56, 57
Life events (see Stressful life events)
Lithium augmentation
dysthymia indications, 19
residual depression, 17
Loss events
anxious depression link, 5
and chronicity, 60
Low back pain, 169

M

Major depression
and attention-deficit/hyperactivity disorder, 198–205
in children, 208–217
age of onset, 211
chronicity, 57, 58
course of, 188
depressive personality relationship, 87–
94
dysthymia relationship, 38, 39, 62
medical model emphasis, 122
as neurotic depression replacement category, 136–139
nosological weaknesses, impact, 119–123
Research Diagnostic Criteria, 134–136

Marital friction, dysthymia link, 11
Marital status, and drug response, 48
Masochism, 5
Maternal depression, 201–203
Medical model, 122
Melancholia
and chronicity, absence of, 61
core signs, 113
drug response, 179
electroconvulsive therapy, 113, 114
psychomotor retardation criterion, 113
Memory, 153
Men, and neurotic depression, 110–112
Minor depression, 183–189
associated psychiatric syndromes, 187
course of, 188, 189
diagnostic criteria, 183, 184
family history, 186, 187
prevalence, 185, 186
sex ratio, 186
social consequences, 185, 186
suicide attempts, 186, 187
Moclobemide
dysthymia response, 20, 40
long-term double-blind study, 40
Monoamine oxidase inhibitors
atypical depression response, 165–169
borderline personality disorder, 178, 179
hysteroid dysphoria response, 174–180
interpersonal sensitivity response, 167–
169
pharmacological dissection, 179
underuse of, 22, 23
Monoamine oxidase levels, 166
"Monocategorical existence," 23
Montgomery–Asberg Depression Rating
Scale, 193
Mood disorders
continuity and chronicity, 54–63
depressive personality association, 89,
90, 92
DSM classification, 10, 11
dysthymia as, 11–15, 25–27
phenomenological constellations, 81–84
Myalgic encephalomyelitis, 154

N

Nefazodone, 17
Neurasthenia, 148–159
and bipolar illness, 4
and chronic fatigue, 6, 7, 148–159
comorbidity, 56

Neurasthenia (continued)
  emphatic listening approach, 7
  minor depression association, 187
  and recurrent brief depression, 187
  symptomatology, 6, 7
Neurotic depression, 3–10, 96–123, 130–144
  characterological features, 8, 9
  clinical heterogeneity, 3–10, 99, 100, 133
  comorbidity, 107, 108
  critical reappraisal, 130–144
  distinctive features, 115–118, 131
  drug response, 118, 177
  DSM dismissal of, 10, 96, 97, 133, 134
    impact of, 119–123
  DSM replacement categories, 136–141
  dysthymia comparison, 96–123
  endogenous depression independence,
    112–114, 119, 121, 132
  follow-up studies, 101–103
  heredity, 108, 109, 118
  ICD-10 replacement categories, 139, 140
  interrater reliability, 133
  misdiagnosis, 2, 3
  need for concept of, 96–123, 141–143
  "personal depression" as alternative, 123
  personality characteristics, 102, 107,
    109–112
    anxiety demarcation, 109–112
    gender differences, 110–112
  psychoanalytic formulation, 99, 100,
    131, 132
  Research Diagnostic Criteria replace-
    ment categories, 134–136
  revival attempts, 141–143
Neuroticism, 110
Newcastle Anxiety–Depressive Diagnostic
  Scale, 110
Noncompliance factors, 22

O

Overtreatment, and residual depression,
  16, 17

P

Pain, 157, 169
Panic symptoms
  dysphoria core pathology, 6
  monoamine oxidase inhibitor response,
    167
  and recurrent brief depression, 187

Parental depression, 201–203
Parental report, 203
Paroxetine, 17
Persistent alterations, 78–81 (see also Resid-
  ual depression)
"Personal depression," 123
Personality Disorder Examination, 70
Personality disorders
  desipramine acute response, 70, 71
  DSM dysthymia classification, 11
Personality traits
  and drug treatment response, 48, 49
  neurotic depression link, 102, 107, 109–
    112
  gender differences, 110–112
Pharmacological dissection
  bipolar diathesis, 21, 222
  chronic dysphorias, 174–180
  dysthymia, 18–22
Phenelzine, 167, 169, 175, 176, 178
Phenomenological constellations
  cluster analysis comparison, 78, 79
  functional psychotic disorders, 75–84
Phenylethylamine, 8
Phobic symptoms, MAOI response, 167
Photophobia, 152
Physician attitudes, 22, 23
Placebo response
  dysthymia long-term study, 40, 41
  episodic depression, 175, 176
Postviral fatigue syndrome
  clinical features, 153, 154
  differential diagnosis, 155–158
Predictive validity, and drug response, 14,
  15
Premorbid characteristics
  chronic depression, 59
  neurotic depression, 109–112
Present State Examination, 78
Primary dysthymia
  classification, 44–46
  comorbidity, 37, 38
  core symptoms, 13
  depressive personality association, 89, 90
  long-term desipramine outcome, 69
  Pittsburgh longitudinal study, children,
    212
  treatment response predictors, 44–51
Pseudo-unipolar depression, 17, 120
Psychiatric and Personal History Schedule,
  78
Psychoanalytic theory, 99, 100, 131, 132
Psychoanalytically oriented psychiatrists, 26
Psychodynamic psychotherapy, 24

Psychoeducational approach, 24, 25
Psychological Impairments Rating Schedule, 78, 81
Psychomotor retardation
  and electroconvulsive therapy, 113, 114
  discriminating power, 113, 118
Psychotherapy
  neurotic depression response, 122
  supportive techniques, 24, 25
Psychotic depression (*see* Endogenous depression)

R

Rapid cycling, 17
Reactive depression
  clinical heterogeneity, 5
  neurotic depression relationship, 99, 100, 118
  psychodynamic formulations, 5
Recovery, dysthymic children, 212, 213, 215
Recurrent brief depression, 183–189
  associated psychiatric syndromes, 187
  course of, 188, 189
  diagnostic criteria, 183, 184
  and dysthymia, 194
  family history, 186, 187
  and neurotic depression, 116, 118
  nosological status, 9, 10
  prevalence, 185, 186, 192, 193
  severity, 193, 194
  sex ratio, 186
  social consequences, 185, 186
  suicide attempts, 186, 187, 191–196
  symptomatology, 9
"Recurrent depressive disorder," 105
Refractory depression (*see* Residual depression)
Rejection sensitivity
  atypical depression, 7, 167
  endogenous depression minimal overlap, 169–171
  monoamine oxidase inhibitor response, 167–169
  operationalization, 168
  and reverse vegetative symptoms, 170, 171
Relapse
  desipramine discontinuation, 69, 70
  and medication withdrawal, 40
Reliability, neurotic depression diagnosis, 133

REM latency
  and pharmacotherapy response, 18, 19
  residual depression, 15
Remission
  definition, 67
  desipramine long-term study, 69, 70
  dysthymic children, 212, 213
  neurotic depression characteristic, 116, 118
  short-term imipramine study, 67, 68
Research Diagnostic Criteria
  neurotic depression replacement categories, 134–136
  usefulness of, 144
Residual depression, 15–18
  causative factors, 15–17
  definition, 78
  and duration of episode, 60
  lithium augmentation in, 17
  phenomenology, 75–84
"Reverse vegetative signs,"
  in atypical depression, 4, 7
  interpersonal sensitivity association, 170, 171
  monoamine oxidase inhibitor response, 166,167
Reversible MAOIs, 22, 23, 199
Ritanserin, 20

S

Sadness criterion, 116, 117
Schizoaffective disorder
  negative social consequences, 81, 82
  phenomenological constellations, 81–84
  residual states, 75–84
Schizophrenia
  negative social consequences, 81, 82
  phenomenological constellations, 81–84
  residual states, 75–84
Schizotypal personality, 90, 92
Selective serotonin reuptake inhibitors (*see also* Fluoxetine)
  dysthymic subgroups response, 46–51
  pharmacological dissection, 179
  physician attitudes, 23
  in residual depression, 17
Self-image, 23
"Self-pitying constellation," 114, 132
Serotonin reuptake inhibitors (*see* Selective serotonin reuptake inhibitors)
Sertraline, 20

Severity of symptoms
  and drug treatment response, 49, 50
  dysthymia criterion, criticism, 104
  ICD-10 staging, 139, 140
  neurotic-endogenous depression, 113
  recurrent brief depression, 193, 194
Sex differences (*see* Gender differences)
Sheehan Disabilities Scales, 36, 39
Sleep EEG, 14
Social Adjustment Scale, 36, 39, 68
Social adjustment
  functional psychoses residual states, 81,
    82
  imipramine response, 68
Social phobia
  dysthymia comorbidity, 37, 38
  and minor depression, 187
  recurrent brief depression association,
    187
"Soft" bipolar signs, 17
Somatic symptoms (*see also* Neurasthenia)
  drug treatment response, 48
  dysthymia comorbidity, 37, 38
  societal influences, 156
Spectrum concept (*see* Continuum concept)
Spontaneous remission, 41
Stereotypes, 23
Stressful life events
  chronicity relationship, 60
  neurotic depression, 99, 100, 106, 107,
    116, 117
    dysthymia comparison, 106, 107
  reactive depression, 5
  residual depression role, 16
Structured Clinical Interview for
  DSM-III-R, 36
Subaffective dysthymia, 11–15
  classification, 11–15, 45
  early- versus late-onset, 46–51
  pharmacological therapy response, 14,
    15, 46–51
  and temperament, 144
Substance use/abuse, 213
Suffering, 12
Suicide/suicide attempts, 191–196
  antidepressant treatment effect, 192, 193
  minor depression, 186, 187
  neurotic depression, 117
  rates of, 191
  recurrent brief depression, 186, 187,
    191–196
Supportive therapy approaches, 24, 25
Symptom severity (*see* Severity of symptoms)

T

Teacher ratings, 203
Temperament
  atypical depression, 7
  chronicity relationship, 59
  dysthymia, 13, 14, 144
  Kraepelin's thesis, 2
  and pharmacotherapy response, 19
  reconceptualization in depression, 144
Tense arousal, 150
"Thoughts of death," 39
Thymoleptics, 14
Thyroid hormones, 150, 151
Tranylcypromine, 40
Treatment failures
  pharmacological factors, 22
  and physician attitudes, 22, 23
Treatment response (*see* Drug response)
Tricyclic antidepressants
  neurotic depression response, 118, 177
  pharmacological dissection strategy, 18–
    20, 177–179
  residual depression cause, 16, 17
Twin studies, 108, 118

U

Undertreatment, 22
Unipolar depression
  DSM-IV elimination of, impact, 119–123
  lithium response, 120
  neurotic depression distinction, 120, 121

V

Vegetative reversal (*see* Reverse vegetative
  signs)
Venlafaxine, 17
Viral mechanisms, 153, 154
Visual scotomata, 152
Vocational adjustment, 68
Vocational guidance, 24, 25

W

Weight gain (*see* Reverse vegetative signs)
Weltschmerz, 12
Women, neurotic depression, 110–112
Work orientation
  as compensatory defense, 24
  in dysthymia, 11, 39
  therapeutic value of, 26